THE
ESTROGEN ALTERNATIVE

WHAT CAN
THE SOY SOLUTION FOR MENOPAUSE
DO FOR ME?

*This life-changing book offers crucial
information on:*

- how soy works to preve

- soy's ability to lessen m
symptoms

- soy's association with l
osteoporosis, heart disease, and cancer

- additional all-natural approaches to
easing menopause, such as herbal
medicine

- recipes, references, and tips for integrating
soy into a healthy lifestyle!

MACHELLE SEIBEL, M.D., is a reproductive endocrinologist at Caritas Norwood Hospital and Professor of Clinical Gynecology at the University of Massachusetts at Worcester. He is also the medical director of Inverness Medical Innovations in Waltham, Massachusetts. He served for nineteen years on the faculty of Harvard Medical School and four years at the Boston University School of Medicine. He has written or edited nine books and authored or co-authored more than two hundred scientific articles. In a national survey of 35,000 doctors he was voted one of the best doctors in America within his specialty.

ODE TO SOY AND HOT FLASHES

Drenched with sweat I wake again
'Cause I'm afraid of estrogen
Can't recall how long it's been
Since I could sleep the night.

Trying soy could do no harm
It stopped the heat, though I'm still warm.
Now I feel my life is charmed
'Cause I can sleep the night.

Experts say, "It's not the same
As estrogen," they all complain.
But it sure helped turn down the flame.
And I can sleep the night!

THE
ESTROGEN
ALTERNATIVE

the
SOY
solution
FOR MENOPAUSE

MACHELLE SEIBEL, M.D.

A FIRESIDE BOOK
Published by Simon & Schuster
New York   London   Toronto   Sydney   Singapore

Every effort has been made to ensure that the information contained in this book is complete and accurate. However, neither the publisher nor the author is engaged in rendering professional advice or services to the individual reader. The ideas, procedures, and suggestions contained in this book are not intended as a substitute for consulting with your physician. All matters regarding health require medical supervision. Neither the author nor the publisher shall be liable or responsible for any loss, injury, or damage allegedly arising from any information or suggestion in this book. The opinions expressed in this book represent the personal views of the author and not of the publisher.

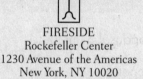

FIRESIDE
Rockefeller Center
1230 Avenue of the Americas
New York, NY 10020

FIRESIDE and colophon are registered trademarks of Simon & Schuster, Inc.

For information regarding special discounts for bulk purchases, please contact Simon & Schuster Special Sales at 1-800-456-6798 or business@simonandschuster.com

Designed by Nancy Singer

Manufactured in the United States of America

10   9   8   7   6   5   4   3   2   1

ISBN 0-7434-2152-3

CONTENTS

ACKNOWLEDGMENTS

No book is written without the help of many people. This book is no exception. In particular, I would like to thank my wife, Dr. Sharon Seibel, for her editorial comments, input, suggestions, and support. I am fortunate to have the help of such a capable person. I would also like to thank my daughter Amy Seibel for constructing some of the figures, Ms. Jane Stephenson for her help with compiling the recipes, and Ms. Mary Everett and Ms. Joanne Casper for reading over the manuscript.

In addition, I would like to express a deep appreciation and gratitude to the many doctors and scientists around the world whose persistent work provided the research and enthusiasm that has brought soy to its current level of understanding. In particular, I would like to thank Doctors Herman Adlercreutz, Stephen Barnes, Tom Clarkson, Mark Messina, Ken Setchell, and Mindy Kurtzer, whose research had a particularly significant impact on my knowledge.

FOREWORD

The Soy Solution for Menopause—The Estrogen Alternative by Dr. Machelle Seibel will help you understand why increasing dietary intake of soy, in both food and supplement forms, can have a major beneficial impact on a woman's transition through the menopausal years. For the past 40 years hormone replacement therapy (HRT) has been used in medicine to treat symptoms of menopause and prevent diseases associated with aging in women. Now modern medicine must re-examine its wholesale dependence on HRT as the magic cure-all for older women.

In July 2002, the *Journal of the American Medical Association* published research concluding that long-term use of HRT may increase cardiovascular and non-cardiovascular risks to menopausal women. Then the National Heart, Lung, and Blood Institute (NHLBI) of the National Institutes of Health (NIH) announced that it canceled a major clinical trial of the risks and benefits of long-term use of the combined hormones estrogen and progestin in healthy menopausal women due to an increased risk of breast cancer and the lack of overall benefit. Thus, the information and advice in this book is highly timely and sensible.

Dr. Seibel has conducted extensive research on the literature surrounding the nutritional and health benefits of soybeans. He states that menopause is not a disease and is a natural progression of a woman's aging process.

The popularity of soy in the U.S. and the West during the past 30 years is phenomenal. I can recall when soy foods could be found in only one of three places: in a small health food store in high-protein powdered drink mixes or vegetarian meat substitutes, in some Chinese restaurants as bean curd (the Asian term *tofu* had not yet caught on), and in the pet food aisle of the grocery or feed store as cheap protein filler. Now, natural foods have become a multi-billion-dollar industry. According to *Functional Foods & Nutraceuticals*, sales of soy foods hit $2.77 billion in 2000, a huge 21% increase from the previous year.

For women and physicians looking for natural alternatives to HRT, there are several herbs and other dietary supplements to consider, as this book points out in Chapter 9, Other Non-Estrogen Approaches to Menopause. The most well-researched herb in this area is black cohosh root (*Actaea racemosa*, syn. *Cimicifuga racemosa*), a plant native to eastern North America long valued by Native Americans. Clinical research in Germany during the past 50 years has documented black cohosh's safe and effective ability to reduce or eliminate some of the symptoms associated with menopause, particularly hot flashes and mood swings.

Another promising herb in this area is red clover (*Trifolium pratense*) that contains some of the same isoflavones found in soy. The growing body of medical research suggests that red clover extract can help treat some of the undesirable symptoms of menopause, and also may help prevent some of the cardiovascular problems and loss of bone density (osteoporosis) associated with menopause.

As Dr. Seibel demonstrates, one of the obvious advantages of soy is that it can be used as both a supplement *and* as a food. Soy is a classic example of the dictum often attributed to the Greek physician Hippocrates, "Your food should be your medicine; your medicine should be your food."

Mark Blumenthal
Founder and Executive Director
American Botanical Council
Editor, HerbalGram
www.herbalgram.org

INTRODUCTION

"I have an earache ... ."

2000 B.C.   Here, eat these beans.

1000 A.D.   Those beans are heathen. Say this prayer.

1880 A.D.   That prayer is superstition. Drink this potion.

1940 A.D.   That potion is snake oil. Take this pill.

1980 A.D.   That pill is ineffective. Take this antibiotic.

2001 A.D.   That antibiotic is artificial. Here, eat these beans.

Anonymous

The 40 million menopausal women in the United States are in a dilemma. Seventy-five percent complain of hot flashes, sexual dysfunction, lack of energy, or other symptoms attributed to the loss of estrogen that comes along with menopause.

Menopause, and the loss of estrogen that comes with it, has also been associated with a higher risk for osteoporosis, heart disease, and diabetes. In fact, heart disease is the leading cause of death for women, killing ten times more women than breast cancer, and osteoporosis will cause bone fractures in 40% of women over the age of 50. That's why many doctors now recommend that their menopausal patients take—or at least consider—hormone replacement therapy (HRT).

And that's the dilemma. Only 9% to 15% of menopausal

women chose to take HRT because they are concerned about the risks and side effects, particularly in light of the articles in July 2002, from the Women's Health Initiative and the National Cancer Institute studies. HRT is associated with an increased likelihood of breast cancer and blood clots. Simply stated, women fear HRT. Many women also experience bloating, weight gain, and abnormal uterine bleeding while taking estrogen. Today's women also tend to avoid synthetic hormones and try a more natural route, especially one that encompasses diet, exercise, and other lifestyle practices.

Here is the good news. There is an excellent alternative to HRT that appears to carry no risk at all. A woman doesn't need a doctor to prescribe it or administer it. All she has to do is add soy products to her diet or take soy supplements. This book explains in simple, understandable language how soy works in the body and how women can get the right kinds and quantities for maximum benefit.

Twenty years ago, practically no scientific papers had been written about soy. But over the past decade, things have changed remarkably. Hundreds of articles are published each year in the world's best journals, touting the health benefits of soy. Now it is well known that soy reduces the severity and number of hot flashes and lowers the risk of osteoporosis, certain cancers, and heart disease.

More than forty well-conducted clinical trials provide compelling evidence that eating soy protein lowers cholesterol. Soy also reduces heart disease by lowering the risk of blood clots and hardening of the arteries (atherosclerosis). These data are so strong that in October 1999 the Food and Drug Administration added soy to its list of foods whose labels can make health claims—in this case, that soy "as part of a diet low in saturated fat and cholesterol, may reduce the risk of heart disease."[1]

Soy is one of the most abundant sources of isoflavones, a type of plant estrogens, or phytoestrogens, that act like real estrogen in the body. While most doctors do not consider soy the same as HRT, many agree that soy is an excellent alternative for the 85% of menopausal women who do not or will not use HRT. In 1999, a consensus among researchers at the annual meeting of the North American Menopause Society concluded: "Of the various classes of phytoestrogens, isoflavones appear to have the most potent estrogenic effects. Isoflavones from soy foods, and in some cases supplements, have beneficial effects on bone mineral density, lipid (cholesterol) profiles, and endothelial (blood vessel) function. Large population-based studies also show inverse relationships between soy isoflavone intake and hormone-replacement cancer risk."[2]

Despite the growing body of evidence that soy is enormously beneficial in lowering the risk of diseases linked to estrogen deficiency, the medical community is still not sure how to relate this information to patients. I have given many lectures across the country at major medical centers, and the most frequent questions asked by doctors are these: "How much soy?" "What form?" "Which supplements?" "How does it work?" Doctors are still learning basic information about soy, so it is not surprising that many perimenopausal and menopausal women ask the same questions. All the confusion and fear surrounding estrogen replacement has created an urgent need for a clear understanding of what to use as an alternative.

This book, throughout, uses simple language to answer questions about how you can use soy to lower your risk of disease and treat the symptoms of menopause. For each health benefit, what form of soy, which soy supplements, how much, how often, and why are all explained. Now you can make your own choices.

The book begins with basic facts about perimenopause and menopause to explain clearly why you must take an active role in disease prevention at this important stage of your life. A chapter explaining HRT, including both its benefits and its risks, follows this. The next chapter explains how soy works in the body to prevent disease. Following chapters focus on the specific health benefits of soy, such as its ability to alleviate menopausal symptoms; its association with lowered risk of osteoporosis, heart disease, and cancer; and its other health benefits. There is a chapter on other non-estrogen approaches for menopause, focusing on herbal medicine and lifestyle. The final chapter includes recipes, references, and tips for integrating soy into your life.

Soy has many health benefits. That is why I wrote *The Soy Solution for Menopause*. I hope you will find this book useful and, after you read it, will want to share it with your mothers, sisters, and friends.

chapter 1

MENOPAUSE AND PERIMENOPAUSE

You have to find out what's good and true and beautiful in your life as it is now. Looking back makes you competitive. And, age is not a competitive issue. . . . The truth is, part of me is every age. I'm a three-year-old, I'm a five-year-old, I'm a thirty-seven-year-old, I'm a fifty-year-old. I've been through all of them and I know what it's like. I delight in being a child when it's appropriate to be a child. I delight in being a wise old man when it's appropriate to be a wise old man. Think of all I can be! I am every age, up to my own.

Morrie Schwartz, from *Tuesdays with Morrie*

I love this passage. It offers so much perspective about aging. In our youth-oriented society, women are often fearful of any label that contains the word "menopause," because it is often presented as a disease or a condition associated with old age. The truth is that for many women, menopause, and the stage of life it represents, are very positive. They no longer fear becoming pregnant and thus have more sexual freedom, and they often have more time and means to enjoy life. A recent Harris poll found that women who turn 50 today view themselves as younger than their parents did at that age, and 51% of 752 postmenopausal women surveyed in 1998 by the North American Menopause

Society reported that they were happier and more fulfilled than they were in their 20s, 30s, and 40s.

UNDERSTANDING THE LINGO

The word "menopause" comes from two Greek words for "month" and "cessation." Menopause is defined by a single event: a woman's last menstrual period, which happens either when a woman's ovaries are removed by surgery (surgical menopause); destroyed by radiation treatments, chemotherapy, or the use of some other drugs (induced menopause); or when her ovaries no longer make enough estrogen to produce a menstrual cycle (natural or spontaneous menopause). It takes one year of waiting after the last period to confirm that it's menopause and not just a very irregular period. "Postmenopause" refers to all the years beyond menopause. Having a hysterectomy (surgical removal of the uterus) will stop menstruation, but it does not cause menopause unless the ovaries are also removed (oophorectomy).

Even though women are living longer than ever before, the age of natural menopause hasn't changed much over the past few centuries. It's still 51.4 years.[1] But menopause any time between the ages of 40 and 55 is normal. Often it occurs around the same time as in one's mother or sister. Premature menopause occurs before age 40, and that happens to about 2% of women.[2] "Perimenopause" means literally "around menopause" and refers to the months and years (up to 10 or 12) preceding menopause plus one year after menopause. Perimenopause is what some women call "being in menopause."

A NATURAL BRIDGE CROSSED OVER BY MANY

Right now, the baby boomers, those enormous numbers of us born in the 1940s and 1950s, are reaching 50. The same people who wanted to change the world in the 1960s are themselves starting to change. Each day, 4,000 American women become menopausal, and their numbers continue to increase: from an estimated 28.7 million women older than 55 in 1990, to 31.2 million in 2000, to a projected 45.9 million by the year 2020. Another 35 million women are currently going through perimenopause. The result of these enormous numbers has been to transform menopause from what author Gail Sheehy called a silent passage into front-page news.

Increasing numbers of books and articles are being published about menopause, and more and more studies are being aimed at women and women's health at this phase of life. The

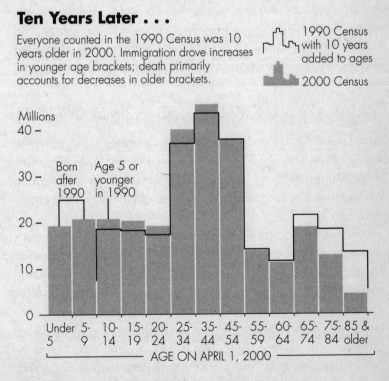

Ten Years Later . . .

Everyone counted in the 1990 Census was 10 years older in 2000. Immigration drove increases in younger age brackets; death primarily accounts for decreases in older brackets.

1990 Census with 10 years added to ages

2000 Census

FIGURE 1-1.   U.S. Census Figures 1990 versus 2000
SOURCE: U.S. Census Bureau.

result is that menopause, often referred to as the change of life, is itself going through a change.

There are important issues for a woman to understand and address as she completes her reproductive years. In her book *Estrogen the Natural Way,* Nina Shandler wrote that "there is a good chance that the vast numbers of female baby boomers are going to grow old—very old."[3] In fact, if a woman reaches 50 without contracting heart disease or cancer, she can expect to live to be 92. Add this to the fact that the fastest-growing age group in America is the 100-plus-year-olds, and it becomes clear that menopause is merely the next phase in a long life, complete with its benefits and its challenges. Realizing that menopause is a natural and inevitable next phase of life is valuable. It allows a person to stop asking the question "How do I stop aging?" and begin asking the question posed by a prominent yogi, Hari Kaur Khalsa: "How do I remain graceful throughout life's challenges?"[4]

WHAT ARE MENOPAUSE AND PERIMENOPAUSE?

Ann Louise Gittleman begins her book *Before the Change* by saying "Peri—what?" She goes on to ask the very question most other 40-plus-year-old women ask as they enter perimenopause and approach menopause: "What on earth is happening to my body?"[5]

Suddenly, an active woman who is used to juggling her work while managing the household, carpooling the kids, and organizing the social calendar starts waking up at 4 A.M. experiencing palpitations in her heart and feeling anxious and depressed. After a while, she is likely to become a little more exhausted and a little more irritable. She notices that she has a shorter attention span and a shorter fuse. Throw in a few mood swings, headaches, and trouble remembering where the car is parked, and suddenly she may be convinced she is having a heart attack, a brain tumor, or a psychiatric problem.

An Aging Population

Increased longevity and the aging of the baby boom generation—age 35 through 54 in the 2000 Census—are the primary reasons for a rising median age.

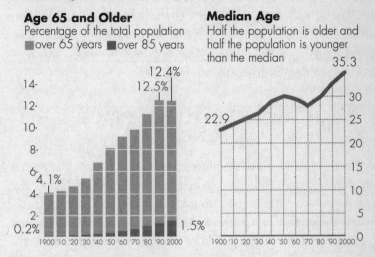

Age 65 and Older
Percentage of the total population
■ over 65 years ■ over 85 years

Median Age
Half the population is older and half the population is younger than the median

FIGURE 1-2.   America Is Growing Older
SOURCE: U.S. Census Bureau.

Many of my perimenopausal patients have already been to another doctor. Her internist might order an electrocardiogram and, seeing that it is normal, offer her Prozac, an often-recommended drug for many of the "female symptoms" associated with perimenopause. The psychiatrist she sees may also suggest an antidepressant or a sleeping tablet. But, if that same 40-plus-year-old woman were to speak with her gynecologist, or a knowledgeable internist or psychiatrist, all of these symptoms would suddenly become recognized as perimenopause.

Unfortunately, probably half of the women seeking medical help for the early symptoms of perimenopause are given a sedative for their anxiety and sent off to the lab for a large battery of tests. Dr. Nancy Lee Teaff, author of *Perimenopause: Preparing for the Change,* said to *New Woman* magazine: "When they first start to appear, perimenopausal symptoms may seem unrelated to each other, and women often treat each problem individually, not seeing the connection until years later. Skipped periods and hot flashes are almost automatically attributed to menopause, but if your first symptom happens to be insomnia, you may spend hours in a therapist's office before it becomes apparent that the problem is primarily hormonal."

HORMONES IN PERIMENOPAUSE AND MENOPAUSE?

At this time, estrogen levels plunge and soar like a wild hormonal roller-coaster ride, and estrogen and progesterone levels no longer work together with precision. In addition to its primary role in stabilizing the uterine lining (the word "progesterone," after all, stems from "pro-gestation"), progesterone also plays a role in a woman's moods by attaching to the same sites in the brain as the neurochemical GABA (gamma amino butyric acid), a hormone secreted into the portal blood (or blood vessels around the pituitary gland) that helps reduce anxiety. This is the same site that Valium attaches to. The impact of having less progesterone clearly varies from one person to another, but the persistent lack of it is believed to play a major role in the mood changes and swings so often experienced by women during perimenopause and menopause.

Hormonally, it's like going through puberty—only backward—and it brings with it some of the same experiences. Menstrual periods become wacky, often being lighter but sometimes heavier, sometimes farther apart or even skipped, but often closer together. And when all of those mood swings and other symptoms kick in, it causes some women to compare perimenopause with a raging case of premenstrual syndrome (PMS). In many ways it is.

As with puberty, there is no one experience, no blueprint for every woman to experience. That is to be expected. People are different before perimenopause; why shouldn't they be different during it? Fortunately, most women won't experience all of the symptoms of perimenopause. But any of them alone or in any combination could be considered typical. Most important of all, perimenopause is only a temporary condition, distressing though it can be. After the hot flashes and PMS, the mood swings and the potential lower self-esteem end, life will improve. Germaine Greer was quoted as saying that her truest self could emerge from the "chrysalis of conditioning" only after menopause had liberated her from her reproductive body.[6]

SYMPTOMS OF PERIMENOPAUSE

- Acne
- Anxiety
- Backache
- Bloating
- Bone loss
- Breast tenderness
- Crying
- Depression
- Facial hair
- Hair loss or thinning
- Headaches
- Heart palpitations
- Hot flashes
- Hypothyroidism
- Insomnia
- Leg cramps
- Lower sexual desire
- Memory problems
- Menstrual cycle irregularities
- Migraines
- Mood swings

- Urine loss
- Vaginal dryness
- Weight gain

FERTILITY DECLINES AS MENOPAUSE APPROACHES

Although a woman plays many important roles throughout her lifetime, as menopause approaches, reproduction often remains an important consideration. Some women are scrambling to have a child; others are hoping not to. In either case, peri-menopause is a time when fertility ebbs and wanes. As a result, estrogen levels fluctuate. Today, reproduction and menopause are interfacing closer and closer because women often delay having children. They are trying to start their careers before they begin a family, or waiting later to marry, or entering a second marriage. During the 1990s, the number of women having a first child before the age of 35 decreased by roughly 22%, and since 1970, there has been a 50% increase in the number of women who have a first child after the age of 35.[7] This trend has led to increasing numbers of advanced reproductive-age women having babies by receiving a donation of eggs from younger women. According to the Society of Assisted Reproductive Technology, this procedure resulted in 2,968 babies being born in 1999.[8] Those who are not planning to have more children wonder when they no longer will have to worry about birth control. The decline in fertility and its accompanying fluctuating estrogen levels are what cause most of the symptoms of perimenopause.

The body works like a thermostat. The pituitary gland, located at the base of the brain, produces follicle-stimulating hormone (FSH). The hormone was given this name because it stimulates the growth and development of follicles—the fluid-filled sac that surrounds each egg. A woman's eggs are produced while she is still in her mother's uterus. During the middle months of pregnancy, a female baby has an enormous number of eggs—about 7 million. During this time of rapid egg production, the female fetus produces high levels of FSH. Over the last half of pregnancy, FSH levels drop sharply and so do the number of eggs. By the infant's birth the number is reduced to 400,000.[9]

These eggs lie dormant within the ovaries until puberty when low FSH levels rise to the normal adult range and each month signal a group of 10 to 20 eggs to mature. The cells around these eggs start producing estrogen, which signals the pituitary gland to stop making more FSH. The estrogen also thickens and prepares the uterine lining in case there is a pregnancy. After a week or so, one of the eggs in the group is selected as the dominant one for that month's group, and a week later it is released in the process called ovulation. The follicle is now called a corpus luteum, and its cells begin to make progesterone as well as estrogen. That stabilizes the uterine lining and prepares it to receive a fertilized egg. If pregnancy does not happen, estrogen and progesterone levels drop over the next two weeks, the old lining is shed as a menstrual period, and the whole process starts again.

Around age 38, eggs are lost from the ovaries at a faster rate,[10] and the symptoms of perimenopause often start about that time. It is estimated that at age 40 a woman has 5,000 to 10,000 eggs left.[11] The eggs that remain are often less responsive to FSH and may not ovulate. I usually explain to patients that the FSH "asks" the ovaries to make an egg develop, but because the ovaries "don't hear it as well," the pituitary gland "speaks louder." Of course, the real reason is that the cells around the eggs produce less estrogen (and less of another hormone called inhibin, whose job it is to keep FSH levels lower), allowing FSH levels to rise.

Most women who conceive easily have FSH levels of 10 milli-international units per milliliter (mIU/ml) or less. FSH levels above 15 mIU/ml suggest that perimenopause is at hand, and levels above 30 to 40 mIU/ml help confirm that menopause has arrived. But FSH levels do fluctuate from month to month, especially in perimenopause, so no one value is foolproof. If you are taking a birth control pill or other estrogen or progesterone medication, it will lower FSH levels. You must stop taking that medication for a week or so to get an accurate measurement of FSH. Of course, if you are in perimenopause and need a contraceptive, keep using one that is nonhormonal (such as a condom or diaphragm) while you wait to check your FSH level.

ESTROGEN—TOO MUCH, TOO LITTLE, TOO MANY?

Mention the word "ovaries" and most people think of reproduction. But the ovaries are much more than two oval containers of eggs. To be sure, reproduction is one of their primary functions. But the ovaries are also highly specialized endocrine glands—organs that produce hormones affecting nearly every organ in a woman's body throughout her lifetime. As with puberty, perimenopause is a time when hormones fluctuate wildly, and that creates some confusion. True, by the time of menopause estrogen levels may drop by as much as 90% from their normal reproductive highs; but early in perimenopause estrogen levels may actually be elevated. That is because the hormones no longer work in synchrony.

One study carefully monitored a perimenopausal woman's hormone levels while she was experiencing periods every 6 weeks.[12] At the beginning of each cycle, her ovaries did not "listen" to her pituitary gland as it sent FSH to summon an egg to develop. As a result, estrogen levels dropped, and her pituitary gland started producing higher levels of FSH. Her body reacted to the low estrogen levels with hot flashes and other symptoms of low estrogen. After a few weeks of being coaxed by higher FSH levels, her ovaries started maturing eggs—even more than

TABLE 1-1. BIRTH CONTROL OPTIONS

	Advantages	Side Effects	Disadvantages
Sterilization Tubal ligation Vasectomy	Safe/highly effective Failure ~5/1,000	Minor surgical procedure	Permanent No protection against HIV and other sexually transmitted diseases
Barrier methods Male condom Female condom Diaphragm Cervical cap Spermicides	All very effective— up to 88%, except spermicides—79% Offer some protection against HIV and sexually transmitted diseases	Possible latex allergy	Must use each time Can break or spill
Birth control pills	Effective—99% safe for healthy nonsmokers; may lower risk of cancer of the uterus and ovary; helps regulate periods in perimenopause	Not recommended for smokers over 35, or a history of breast cancer or jaundice. Weight gain, breast tenderness, nausea, and spotting possible. May deplete B complex vitamins	No protection against HIV or sexually transmitted diseases; some risk of blood clots, especially in smokers; lowers FSH levels
Progesterone Injections (Depo-provera) Implant (Norplant)	Effective—99%; Single injection lasts 3 months Implants last up to 5 years and are reversible when removed	Weight gain and menstrual cycle changes, headaches, nervousness, dizziness, acne, risk of blood clots Implant can cause scars because requires surgery to remove	No protection against HIV or sexually transmitted diseases Shot can take 12–18 months for return of fertility
Intrauterine device (IUD)	Highly effective— 99%, up to 10 years; reversible when removed, newer devices safer with no increased risk of pelvic infection	Cramping, spotting, heavier periods; not recommended for history of pelvic infection, abnormal genital bleeding, or anemia	Must check for string regularly to see if still in place No protection against HIV or sexually transmitted diseases
Natural family planning Rhythm Withdrawal Persona	No cost or preparation for rhythm or withdrawal	None	No protection against HIV or sexually transmitted diseases Difficult to use with irregular cycles of perimenopause

SOURCE: Modified from *Menopause Guidebook*, North American Menopause Society, 1998: 4–5 (www.menopause.org).

usual—causing a large burst of estrogen to enter her bloodstream. The woman went from having hot flashes to having breast tenderness and bloating—symptoms of too much estrogen. All this took place within the same menstrual cycle. This particular woman went on to ovulate, make progesterone, and have a period two weeks later. However, because the eggs of a perimenopausal woman are typically resistant to FSH, sometimes no egg is released and progesterone is not produced. This study helps explain why early in perimenopause it may not be more estrogen that is needed. There may already be more than enough. But because you will not always be ovulating, it may be progesterone and not estrogen that is too low.

To add to the confusion, there are three major estrogens, not just one. Their names are estrone (E1), estradiol (E2), and estriol (E3). The 1, 2, and 3 are used to let us know how many OH molecules are on the estrogen. The suffix one stands for one OH molecule, diol for two molecules, and triol for three. Most of the estradiol is made in the ovaries. But estrone is manufactured primarily in the body's fat cells by a process called aromatization. The enzyme aromatase takes androgen hormones (see section Other Hormones That Change with Menopause) and aromatizes or converts them into estrone. Just as you might guess, women who have more fat on their bodies make more estrone. More estrone is good news for some women because it may lower the symptoms of menopause, but it is also a major reason why women who are significantly overweight have a higher risk of uterine cancer—three times higher if they are 25 to 50 pounds overweight and nine times higher if they are more than 50 pounds overweight. At the opposite extreme, women who are too thin and who have too little fat on their bodies may stop having periods altogether, because their body does not produce enough estrogen.

Estradiol is the major estrogen produced by the ovaries before menopause. It is also the most potent—12 times more than estrone and 80 times more than estriol. After menopause, estradiol levels drop by as much as 90% because almost all of it comes from the ovaries, and they stop making it. Estrone levels drop by as much as one third as the ovaries stop making it. But estrone continues to be made in the body's fat tissue, and obese women (more than 20% over ideal body weight) can make up to 40% more estrogen than non-obese women.[13] Other organs, including the brain, muscles, lungs, skin, and bone marrow, also are able to convert androgens into estrone. The body makes only very small amounts of estriol, except during pregnancy when the placenta increases production of the hormone by more than a thousandfold. In contrast to estradiol and estrone, estriol does not appear to be linked with any increased risk of cancer and, in fact, may be protective against it.

OTHER HORMONES THAT CHANGE WITH MENOPAUSE

Testosterone and androstenedione are two other hormones that change during and after menopause. These two hormones, androgens, are so-called male hormones. Of course, these hormones are present in both men and women, but women have lower levels than men, just as men have lower estrogen levels than women. After menopause, testosterone levels drop by as much as 28%. It happens in all women, but it happens faster and to a greater extent in women who have had their ovaries removed.[14]

Before menopause, about 25% of testosterone is made in the ovaries. Another 25% comes from the adrenal glands, and the remaining half comes from the body's fat cells. After menopause, the percentages change. One fourth is still produced in the adrenal glands, but the ovaries now produce 40% and the fat cells make 35%. One real benefit of keeping one's ovaries is that testosterone levels remain higher, which helps lessen the symptoms of perimenopause and menopause. As Dr. Susan Love's *Hormone Book* puts it, "The menopausal ovary is neither failing nor useless. It's simply beginning to shift from its reproductive to its maintenance function. In midlife it is doing exactly what many people do—it's changing careers."[15]

After menopause, the adrenal glands slowly begin to produce lesser amounts of androstenedione. Because the drop in testosterone and androstenedione happen slowly, naturally postmenopausal women usually do not have a loss of libido. If there is a loss of libido and testosterone levels are not low, giving testosterone probably will not make it better. Loss of libido must be looked for in other causes. But if testosterone levels are lower than expected, testosterone replacement can make a difference.

REGULAR PHYSICAL EXAMS ARE KEY

So many things change during perimenopause and menopause that it can be difficult to know what is normal and what is not. Every day can be a new experience—not necessarily a bad one. That is why it is so important to keep a close eye on your health. With so many years likely to be ahead of you, staying well

TABLE 1-2. FACTORS AFFECTING AGE OF MENOPAUSE

Later Onset	Earlier Onset
Larger body mass	Smoking
Delivering many babies	Not delivering a baby
	Medically treated depression
	Toxic chemical exposure
	Childhood cancer treated with pelvic radiation or certain chemotherapy

becomes much wiser than trying to get well. Here are some things that you and your doctor should check regularly:

- **Blood glucose test** to screen for diabetes or hypoglycemia; 18 million Americans have it, and another 6 million don't realize that they do.
- **Blood pressure** test to screen for high blood pressure.
- **Breast exam** each month by you and each year by your doctor; mammograms every year if you have a strong family history of breast cancer and every two if you do not.
- **Cholesterol profile** to screen for a major risk factor for heart disease. High levels of cholesterol (above 200 milligrams per deciliter or 5.18 millimoles per liter) or LDL (low-density lipoprotein, "bad cholesterol") above 130 significantly increase the risk of heart disease. Soy protein has been approved by the Food and Drug Administration as being able to lower cholesterol levels if taken with a good diet and a healthy lifestyle.
- **Complete blood count (CBC)** to screen for anemia and make certain your blood components are normal.
- **Dental and eye care**—Remember teeth are bones and need protection from osteoporosis; soy may help to maintain bone health by slowing the loss of calcium.
- **Immunizations** are recommended every 10 years for tetanus and diphtheria; older or infirm people need flu shots every year.
- **Pelvic exam** each year by a gynecologist, skilled internist, or family practitioner, including a Papanicolaou smear (Pap smear) to check for cancer of the cervix (opening of the uterus) and rectal exam to screen for occult blood (guaiac test)—a test for colon cancer. Discuss getting an ultrasound of the ovaries if there is a family history of ovarian cancer. I would also recommend an ultrasound of the ovaries if there is a strong family history of breast cancer, because there is a genetic link between breast cancer and ovarian cancer.

- **Skin cancer exam**—Check the skin of the entire body every 3 years to screen for malignant melanoma, the deadliest form of skin cancer. People with a family history of skin cancer and those who have a lot of moles, or a history of a blistering sunburn as a child, should check more often.
- **Urinalysis** for kidney disorders and urinary tract infections as well as screening for other diseases such as diabetes by finding high levels of glucose in the urine.

THINGS TO CHECK FOR DURING AND AFTER MENOPAUSE
Changes in the Menstrual Cycle

Even if it starts out subtly, it is almost inevitable that menstrual cycles will become irregular during perimenopause and beyond. More than 70% of women will experience irregular menstrual cycles in their 40s. As mentioned earlier, these irregularities may be longer cycles or shorter cycles, heavier or lighter cycles, increased bleeding or skipped bleeding. Most of the time the "abnormal" bleeding will turn out to be normal, but it's important to be certain. Here are some of the things you and your doctor should watch out for:

- **Pregnancy**—Impossible? No! If you are not menopausal it can still happen. Every year or so, at least one of my perimenopausal patients comes in having not had a period in a few months and thinks she may finally be in menopause—except that she feels pregnant. And she is. Even women who have been infertile and haven't used birth control for years must consider pregnancy as a possible cause of abnormal bleeding or absent periods.
- **Fibroids**—These are benign tumors that grow in or on the uterus. I often describe them as being like a knot in a pine

tree. Fibroids prevent the muscles of the uterus from squeezing the blood vessels that pass through it, so bleeding continues after the expected time. Usually they do not cause any symptoms, but they can cause pain during intercourse, low back pain, frequent urination, or menstrual cramps.

- **Precancer, cancer, and polyps**—When the uterine lining grows excessively, it can go through changes that lead to cancer. This is called hyperplasia. Polyps are also a type of tissue buildup of the lining. They are actually fleshy growths in the lining of the uterus. It takes about ten years for hyperplasia to turn into cancer. That is why it is so important to find out the cause of abnormal bleeding early. It helps to ensure a cure.

FINDING OUT WHY

Most of the time I can tell whether irregular bleeding is a problem just by listening to my patient's history. But it is difficult to be absolutely certain that irregular bleeding is normal, or at least not a cause for concern. Most of the time it becomes necessary to find the reason for the bleeding. Several methods can be used, and each has its benefits:

- **Dilatation and curettage (D&C)**—The cervix or neck of the uterus is stretched slightly (dilated) and a small amount of the lining is scraped out (curettage) and looked at under the microscope by a pathologist. A D&C is usually performed with anesthesia in an operating room. An endometrial biopsy is a "mini" D&C commonly performed in the office. The instruments are small, and local anesthesia or sometimes no anesthesia is needed.
- **Hysteroscopy**—"Hystero" is the Greek root for uterus, so a hysteroscopy uses a tiny telescope to look inside the uterus.

Any abnormality can be seen and tested. The newer hysteroscopes are so small that the procedure can be done in the office, usually without needing anesthesia.

- **Transvaginal ultrasound**—A small probe the size of a thumb is inserted into the vagina to view the pelvic organs, using sound waves. The procedure is painless, and there is no radiation. This procedure can be used only as a screen and may miss small abnormalities. Sometimes a small amount of saline (about a tablespoon) is injected into the uterus to help outline small abnormalities and the transvaginal ultrasound probe is then used. This is called a sonohysterogram.

CHOOSING A TREATMENT

As with every other medical problem, treatment depends in part on the cause and in part on the preferences of the patient, her age, and her general health. Take the time to discuss all the treatment choices with your doctor, and make sure you understand the benefits and risks of each. The major treatments for menstrual abnormalities can be divided into two categories: medications and surgery.

Medications

Once it's clear that abnormal bleeding is due to a hormonal imbalance and not a more serious problem, correcting the imbalance will solve the problem. The most important point in choosing the treatment is understanding which hormone is out of balance. Sometimes that means prescribing estrogen, sometimes progesterone, and sometimes a combination of the two. Other medications such as Lupron (leuprolide acetate) can also be used for short periods of time. This medication turns off the pituitary gland and causes a reversible medical menopause.

Surgery

Several types of surgery can be used to treat abnormal bleeding. I believe there are only three important things a surgeon must know: (1) when an operation is necessary, (2) which operation to perform, and (3) when to stop operating. If you are comfortable that your gynecologist has the answers to these questions, you will have chosen both the right operation and the right person to perform it. The most common surgeries are these:

- **D&C**—Not only a way to diagnose but many times can also treat abnormal uterine bleeding by giving the lining a fresh start.
- **Operative hysteroscopy**—This is similar to the hysteroscopy used to diagnose abnormal bleeding. The main difference is that the telescope is larger so surgical instruments can pass through it. Either a laser or an electrical loop is used to remove polyps or fibroids bulging into the uterus. Newer instruments have been developed that can destroy the entire uterine lining, the endometrium, by freezing or cauterizing it. The procedure is called endometrial ablation, and it permanently stops all bleeding in 50% of women. It also removes any future chance for pregnancy. About 40% of women will continue to have light periods because some of the lining cells are not destroyed, and 10% of women will not be helped at all.
- **Laparoscopy**—This is called the "belly button" operation. A telescope the size of a ballpoint pen is inserted into the abdomen through a half-inch incision under the umbilicus. Abnormalities on the outside of the uterus or the ovaries can be seen and—depending on the skill of the surgeon and how major the problem—corrected at the same time. Usually this is same-day surgery.
- **Hysterectomy**—This operation involves removal of the entire uterus. It will stop all menstrual bleeding and makes it no longer possible to carry a baby, but it will not cause

menopause unless both ovaries are also removed (bilateral oophorectomy). One third of all women in the United States will have had a hysterectomy and bilateral oophorectomy before they are 60. Many women who have had a hysterectomy report that they feel better, their sex life has improved, and they are happy with their choice. But be sure to discuss your other options. Once the uterus has been removed, there is no going back. Fibroids can be removed by laparoscopy and through an abdominal incision, saving the uterus. Even a hysterectomy done to remove a uterus that is dropping or associated with urine loss can often be avoided by choosing other procedures. When a woman is clear that her hysterectomy is necessary and she and her partner both agree the operation is the correct choice for them, sexual intercourse is usually not affected.[16] Remember the three questions I raised earlier, and be certain that hysterectomy is the right choice for you.

Urinary Tract Problems

Did you know that more adult absorption pads, such as Depends, are sold each year than disposable diapers? Urinary tract problems are a major problem for the American population and one of the most embarrassing aspects of aging. Men with an enlarged prostate gland (which up to 50% of men have after age 50) or who have had surgery to treat prostate cancer may involuntarily lose their urine from time to time. But the involuntary loss of urine (incontinence) is definitely a problem more common in women than in men.[17] Half of all menopausal women have at least some involuntary urine loss, and 25% need surgery to correct it. That is because the urethra—the tube that carries urine from the bladder out of the body—is much shorter in women than in men. Added to that fact is the wear and tear of childbirth, which can weaken the pelvic muscles and the fascia, the sheath that reinforces and additionally supports the ure-thra.[18] That is why women who have had children are more likely to have urine loss than those who have not.

Menopause also contributes to urinary tract problems because the lining of the urethra, the fascia, and the pelvic mus-cles that surround them are sensitive to estrogen and may weaken when estrogen levels decline. All of this can lead to leak-age of urine. There are several types of incontinence. One, called urge incontinence, affects about 10% of postmenopausal women. If you have this problem, you will feel a strong need to urinate that comes on very quickly. Even though you tighten up all your pelvic muscles, you may not be able to get to the toilet in time to prevent leakage because you cannot control the bladder and keep the urine in. You might always feel that you have to go, only to find out you make very little urine.

Another type of incontinence, stress incontinence, is much more common. Menopause contributes to this problem, but stretching and tearing of the pelvic muscles during childbirth definitely sets the stage. The reduced muscle tone causes the urethra to sag. When pressure builds up in the abdomen, or your organs put pressure on your bladder, a small amount of urine may escape. You may notice urine loss when you cough, sneeze, laugh, jump, or lift. That is what makes it such an incredible nui-sance and so embarrassing—it can occur at any time.

Overflow incontinence, a third type, happens when more urine collects in the bladder than the bladder can hold. The excess urine leaks out. It can be caused by blockage of the uri-nary tract or nerve damage caused by conditions such as dia-betes, stroke, or injury. It is also common in men who have an enlarged prostate gland.

Functional incontinence is not really a medical problem. It happens to people who cannot move quickly, who have eye prob-lems, or who suffer from confusion or memory loss. They simply can't get to the bathroom in time.

The North American Menopause Society's *Menopause Guidebook* points out that infection of the bladder (cystitis), other medical conditions such as multiple sclerosis, certain prescription drugs such as diuretics and some tranquilizers, and smoking and drinking alcohol and caffeine, which irritate the bladder, make incontinence worse.[19]

FIRST, FIND THE CAUSE

Treating urinary tract problems can be tricky. Always take the time to find out what is causing your problem; otherwise, you are likely to choose the wrong treatment, and it will not work. A complete urinalysis and a pelvic exam are basic, and specialized studies of the bladder are often also needed. The American Medical Association's *Essential Guide to Menopause* lists medications such as antihypertensives and antidepressants; foods such as sugar, coffee, alcohol, artificial sweeteners, and spicy dishes; and smoking as contributors to incontinence if the muscles are already weakened.[20]

Many gynecologists are able to determine the cause of your urinary tract problem and treat it. But if he or she is not, there is a new subspecialty of gynecologists called urogynecologists. After completing their training in gynecology and obstetrics, these specialists spend an additional three years learning about these types of problems. Some urologists also focus on female urology. If you are not sure of the cause of the problem, are unhappy with your treatment options, or want a second opinion, make an appointment to see one of these folks.

CHOOSING A TREATMENT

Twenty years ago, the options for treating many types of urinary tract problems were limited. The only choice offered was a hysterectomy. Today, there are many more options to consider. Here are some of the more common ones:

- **Bladder training**—This approach teaches you to urinate only at scheduled times and to wait longer between trips to the bathroom. Start by going to the bathroom every 30 to 60 minutes while you are awake, even if you don't have to go. After about one week, slowly increase the time interval by 30 minutes every week. Eventually you can modify how often you have to go by training your bladder to wait at least 4 hours. Remember first to be certain that you do not have an infection.

- **Kegel exercises**—Although these exercises were first described in the medical literature by Dr. Kegel, a similar yoga exercise known as the *root lock* has been around for centuries. Kegel exercises can improve the symptoms of urinary loss by 25% to 50%. Kegel exercises strengthen pelvic muscles, and, like other muscle-building exercises, they work best if you perform a lot of repetitions. Start them the next time you go to the bathroom by squeezing off the urine flow and holding it for up to 10 seconds. You can also place a finger inside your vagina and tighten up on it. Once you know which muscles to squeeze, you do not have to be in the bathroom. You can do Kegel exercises anywhere at any time—in the car, sitting on the couch watching television, or typing at your computer. Start slowly, doing two sets of 10 contractions each, twice a day. Over the course of a month, try to do this exercise 6 to 10 times every hour or two hours each day. By the end of a month, you should begin to notice a difference. Learning how to time a pelvic muscle contraction to occur during a cough may eliminate stress incontinence during that cough.[21] Another benefit of Kegel exercises is that they may improve sexual satisfaction, because those pelvic muscles are the same ones used during sexual intercourse.

- **Medications**—Estrogen has been helpful in improving the symptoms of incontinence in 40% to 70% of women. I have found that estrogen cream (half an applicator) works better than either tablets or patches for this particular problem. I suggest using it every other day for two weeks and then once or twice a week after that. After three months, the tissue usually has regained much of its strength and the medication can be stopped. Performing Kegel exercises during the same time period really helps. If you try this approach, do not be surprised if your breasts and nipples feel fuller or even tingle, because some of the estrogen will be absorbed into your bloodstream. Medications called antimuscarinic (examples are oxybutynin and tolterodine[22]) can also help if the problem is caused by abnormal bladder contractions.[23] If you have certain medical conditions such as glaucoma, high blood pressure, or heart disease, these medications may not be right for you. For infection, antibiotics are the first-line treatment.

- **Pessary**—This is a doughnutlike plastic ring that fits into the vagina like a diaphragm to offer added support for the bladder when the pelvic muscles are weak. It is not for everyone but it is worth a try before having surgery. Another option that works along the same lines is a tampon. Placing one in to support the bladder works as well as a pessary, or even better, for some women. If you do try the tampon approach, remember to change it often to prevent toxic shock syndrome.[24]

- **Special devices**—New devices are constantly coming onto the market to block or capture urine leakage. They include absorbent products, external urine collection devices, and different types of catheters.

- **Biofeedback**—These devices use mild electrical stimulation to train the bladder muscles when and how to squeeze. In a way, such a device is a personal trainer for Kegel exercises.

- **Surgery**—Many new operations have been developed to support the bladder and improve or correct incontinence.

You definitely do not need to have a hysterectomy unless there are other reasons to consider it. Most of these alternative operations can be performed as same-day surgeries. Some use laparoscopy; others, only small incisions. They all are designed to repair tears in the support tissue and/or support the urethra.[25]

Changes in Desire

Many years ago I was taking care of a lovely septuagenarian whose husband had died a decade earlier. She had finally entered into a new relationship and had come to me for surgery to correct her dropped bladder and uterus, which were causing her some discomfort. She said to me, "You know, Doctor, I really need to get this fixed. My new friend is interested in more than just my cooking."

Sex and sexuality is a very important part of every person's well-being. I explain to my patients any surgical procedure that might affect their sexual desire, and we discuss sexual desire as part of their annual exams. Sometimes the discussion concerns a loss of libido. My conversations with my patients agree with the report of the *Second Task Force on Female Sexuality During the Menopause,* which ranked reduced sexual desire (lack of sexual fantasies, reduced or absent desire for sexual activities, or lack of reception to sexual initiation) as the most common female sexual complaint.[26] However, women generally continue to be sexually active as long as they remain healthy and, as the *Second Task Force on Sexuality During the Menopause* points out, as long as they continue to have an available partner. Fear of losing a partner often leads to discussions about a spouse who has had a heart attack and is afraid to have sex. Sometimes the spouse has started using Viagra to help his libido and in the process "overcorrected" the problem, making him more interested in sex than his wife is. It is always risky to generalize, but for many women, the sexual drive tends to be motivated by the wish for intimacy. The sexual drive of men is often driven by fantasy and is focused on intercourse and orgasm. Patients often tell me they are no longer worried about contraception and the demands of children, and they feel freer and unburdened, but their vagina is dry and becomes irritated with intercourse. Painful intercourse is one of the main reasons for the decline in sexual activity among menopausal patients. Fortunately, it's a problem that can usually be diagnosed during the pelvic exam.

Despite all the talk about Viagra, I believe the most important sex organ is the brain. When either men or women between the ages of 45 and 59 were asked what would improve their sex lives, the main factors were less stress and more free time. Factors like the quality of the relationship before menopause, the quality of one's health, how one feels about oneself, and the expectations one has of menopause will all play an important role in how sexual function will change after menopause. That is why it is so important not to forget to add a little romance. Of course, age itself will slowly have an effect on frequency and the level of interest. For women between the ages of 60 and 74 years, better health for their partners was the key issue to making things better. After age 75, the main deterrent to having a healthy sex life is lack of a partner. Among those 85 years of age or older, there are 44 men for every 100 women.[27] But things do not halt abruptly, and every individual is different.

Common complaints like vaginal dryness are caused by the body's reduced estrogen levels. As one of my patients put it, "I'm so uncomfortable it's just not worth it." Simply taking more time with more foreplay may be enough to solve the problem. Vitamin E can also add lubrication and heal thinned vaginal tissue. Just take one of those gel tablets out of the bottle, prick it, and rub the vitamin E inside your vagina or on the surrounding skin (the vulva). Vaginal moisturizers like Replens are also helpful. It is also worthwhile to start a steady diet of soy. Some, but not all, studies have shown that soy is helpful in changing the vagina to a more premenopausal state. If that does not work, as Claudia Kalb wrote in *Newsweek*: "What could be more logical than treating sex problems with sex hormones?"[28] Estrogen—and possibly testosterone if levels are low—will solve this problem. Both these hormones appear to influence sexual desire through a positive effect on the brain.

Changes in Metabolism Are the Norm

Older adults are not simply a more aged version of younger adults.[29] Menopause and aging in general are associated with changes in metabolism. In fact, metabolism first starts to slow down during your 30s, causing the percentage of lean muscle in your body to decrease while fat increases. During your 40s, things change even more. Your basal metabolic rate drops by 4% to 5% each decade, making it increasingly more essential to make healthy dietary choices such as soy and to keep exercising. By the time you reach your 50s, your body needs 50 fewer calories each day than you did in your 40s in order not to gain weight. That is why it is so easy for pounds to sneak up on you if you waste your calories on empty ones.

Your 60s continue along the same line, with most of any added weight finding its home in the abdominal area. Increasing girth adds to the risk of high blood pressure and diabetes. It is really important during this decade to keep exercising. Do not forget to consider weight training. Not only can it help to fight off medical risks by burning off unwanted calories, but also it can keep up your muscle strength and tone. By your 70s, loss of muscle strength and tone are common, as are losses of bone density. Some of this loss is due to a decrease in dietary intake or a loss in appetite.

I think this point is important, and understanding it may be helpful. As we age we become more and more creatures of habit, even when it comes to food. A report in the *Journal of the American Medical Association* emphasized this point. After a period of deliberate overfeeding, young men reduced their voluntary intake of food, but elderly men continued to over-feed themselves. Conversely, after a period of enforced under-feeding, young men increased their energy intake to make up for what they had lost, whereas elderly men continued to underfeed themselves for up to 10 days.[30] As the authors point out, if an older person goes through a period of energy restric-tion, such as that caused by illness or depression, we can't assume that he or she will quickly start eating again once the problem passes. We have to also keep in mind that between 30% and 50% of women 65 years and older live alone and are less likely to cook for themselves and more likely to either not eat or go out and eat higher-calorie meals. Such situations can modify eating habits and have a major impact on a person's nutrition.

Other factors also play a role. Up to 30% of people over age 60 secrete less acid into the stomach, a condition known as hypochlorhydria.[31] This allows more of the bacteria swallowed into the stomach to survive, and that changes the digestion of sugar. Instead of being digested just as it passes out of the stomach, sugars pass into the colon, where they ferment and cause more gas to form. These changes affect the absorption of riboflavin and vitamins B_6, B_{12}, and D. In addition to reduced absorption, an extra amount of vitamin D is also needed because the skin of menopausal women (and men of compara-ble age) is less able to synthesize it, and the kidneys are less able to turn 25-hydroxyvitamin D into the active 1,25-dihy-droxy form that is needed. Since vitamin D is needed for the body to absorb calcium, less calcium gets absorbed as well. Add to this the fact that across all ages, nearly 75% of women consume too little calcium to maintain strong bones. Eating well helps to offset these problems. Exercise is important for maintaining flexibility, which can help prevent falls, and for maintaining strength.

How do doctors determine whether a person is overweight? We use a tool called the body mass index (BMI). It considers your weight and your height together. Look down the first column of the chart to find your height, and then scan across to your weight. Your body mass index is the number on top of that column. A body mass index below 25 is the goal; one that exceeds 25 indicates overweight, and BMIs above 30 are categorized as obese.

TABLE 1-3. BODY MASS INDEX

	21	22	23	24	25	26	27	28	29	30
5'0"	107	112	118	123	128	133	138	143	148	153
5'1"	111	116	122	127	132	137	143	148	153	158
5'2"	115	120	126	131	136	142	147	153	158	164
5'3"	118	124	130	135	141	146	152	158	163	169
5'4"	122	128	134	140	145	151	157	163	169	174
5'5"	126	132	138	144	150	156	162	168	174	180
5'6"	130	136	142	148	155	161	167	173	179	186
5'7"	134	140	146	153	159	166	172	178	185	191
5'8"	138	144	151	158	164	171	177	184	190	197
5'9"	142	149	155	162	169	176	182	189	196	203
5'10"	146	153	160	167	174	181	188	195	202	207
5'11"	150	157	165	172	179	186	193	200	208	215

When exercising, the goal is to choose a level that will cause your heart to beat at 60% to 75% of its maximum capacity. If you do this, you will achieve maximum cardiovascular benefit without overtaxing your heart. The desired heart rate changes with age and health. Discuss what is an ideal heart rate for you with your doctor. The table below shows an advisable range.

TABLE 1-4. TARGET HEART RATE

Age	Beats per Minute
20	120–160
25	117–156
30	114–152
35	111–148
40	108–144
45	105–140
50	102–136
55	99–132
60	96–128
65	93–124
70	90–120

Psychological Changes

There are many myths about the mental state of women going through menopause. But there are also some truths. For instance, depression strikes two women for every man. People who are depressed are more than twice as likely to smoke as the general population.[32] There are also gender differences between how men and women perceive emotions. Dr. Mark George of the National Institute of Mental Health performed PET (positron emission tomography) scans on both male and female subjects while asking them to conjure up their saddest memory. The test maps the flow of blood in areas of the brain that are at work during a given time. He found that during memories of strong emotion the total area of women's brains that were active was eight times larger than the total active area of men's brains. This showed a very different experience between the genders.

There are other differences as well. According to scientists at McGill University, serotonin production is 53% higher in men's brains than in women's. Serotonin is the brain chemical that is believed to be lower in people who suffer from depression than in nondepressed individuals. A large number of drugs, categorized as selective serotonin reuptake inhibitors (SSRIs), increase serotonin levels in the brain. Sales of these medications, for example Prozac, Zoloft, Paxil, Lovan, and Luvox, are brisk because more than 17% of all Americans are likely to suffer at least one episode of major depression in their lifetime.

While all of this is important, none of it happens because of menopause. Despite the myths and stories of the middle-aged woman suddenly becoming depressed or a shrew, the truth is quite to the contrary. Sure, there are mood swings, and perimenopausal women often describe PMS-type symptoms. Some women clearly are more sensitive to loss of estrogen than others. But published reports on more than 13,000 perimenopausal women in Norway,[33] Canada,[34] and Massachusetts[35] suggest there is no increase in psychological symptoms. That is not to say that a woman who is depressed before perimenopause will not feel even sadder going through menopause, or if perimenopause is long and symptomatic some feelings of depression will not creep in. But the experience varies widely and will depend a great deal on the individual.

Sometimes we are called the "sandwich generation." We are sandwiched in between our children who demand and need our time and attention and our aging parents who need us as well. Real life is stressful without menopause, and different people have different coping skills. If perimenopause or menopause is creating a stressful life for you, it is treatable. Seek the help of a therapist. Also discuss the problem with your family doctor. Symptoms such as depression and mood swings can also be due to diet and hypoglycemia (low blood sugar) as well as hormonal fluxes. Thyroid disease is also more common in women than in men and is affected by changing estrogen levels, diet, and exercise. Both hypoglycemia and thyroid disease can have a major effect on mood, and they can be treated.

Osteoporosis

Osteoporosis or thinning of the bones affects 28 million Americans, 80% of whom are women (see Chapter 5). About 38% of African-Americans have bone loss that can lead to osteoporosis compared with 50% and more among Caucasians, Hispanics, and Asians. Bone loss is one of the most important changes that occur with menopause, because not only can it cause unsightly physical changes, such as a dowager's hump and loss of height (sometimes more than 2 inches), it can also lead to a broken hip—a life-threatening condition.

Women should get a bone-density test as menopause approaches. A bone-density test has only 10% of the radiation that occurs in a routine chest X-ray and it will diagnose the problem. In addition, here are some other things that you can do to help:

- Quit smoking.
- Exercise 30 minutes three to five times a week—jogging, jumping rope, walking briskly, or lifting weights can boost bone density 3% to 5% a year.
- Avoid excessive alcohol.
- Take 1,200 milligrams (mg) of calcium, 400–800 international units (IU) of vitamin D, and 400 mg of magnesium daily.
- Eat healthy—in Chapter 5 I'll explain how eating soy can help lower your risk for osteoporosis and keep your bones healthy.

Cancer

"You have cancer" are probably the three most dreaded words in the English language. More than 1,500 people in the United States die each day from this dreaded disease. As Dartmouth biochemist Constance Brinckerhoff told *Newsweek* magazine, "In an instant your world is turned upside down, and no matter what follows, it will never be exactly the same." Menopause does not increase the risk of cancer, but cancer rates do tend to increase with age, which is why it is so important to eat well, live well, and have regular checkups.

Breast cancer is the most commonly diagnosed malignancy in American women. In 2000, 30% of all new female cancer cases in the United States, about 182,800, were breast cancer cases.[36] Fortunately, the annual death toll is much lower (41,943 or 15% of all cancer deaths in 1999). Of the breast cancers diagnosed, 42,600 will be in situ, meaning local and not spread. Although lung cancer (61,922 or 25% of all cancer deaths in 1999) and heart disease (over 505,000 deaths) are responsible for many more deaths, neither instills the intense fear and insecurity of breast cancer.

In the past two years, I have accompanied both my mother and my wife into the hospital for a breast biopsy. Both had regular checkups and regular mammograms and lead healthy lives. Both had new specks of calcium on their mammograms. My mother's turned out to be a small in situ cancer—one that had not spread. There is a 97% chance that she is cured. My wife's turned out to be benign. In both instances, waiting for the results were the longest days of our lives. We were very fortunate.

Breast cancer rates have remained approximately level in the 1990s. Nearly half the cases occur in women 65 years and older. Less than 10% of cases occur in women under 40 in the United States and Canada, and 15% occur in women under 50. According to Dr. Susan Love, a noted breast cancer surgeon, the median age for breast cancer is 69. It is a diagnosis that will kill approximately one third of the women diagnosed with it. If you are 50 years old, your lifetime probability of getting breast cancer is 10% and the chance of dying of the disease is 3%.[37] Here is a breakdown of breast cancer risk by age:

TABLE 1-5. BREAST CANCER RISK BY AGE

Age	Percentage
50	2
60	4–5
70	7
80	9–10

SOURCE: American Cancer Society (www.cancer.org).

The American Cancer Society breaks things down a little differently. The probability of developing invasive cancer (this is cancer that has begun to spread and is the kind that can kill you) compared to some of the other most common cancers is:

TABLE 1-6. CANCER RISK BY AGE

Type of Cancer	Birth to 39 (%)	40 to 59 (%)	60 to 79 (%)	Birth to Death
Breast	0.43 (1 in 235)	4.06 (1 in 25)	6.88 (1 in 15)	12.56 (1 in 8)
Colon/ Rectum	0.05 (1 in 1,947)	0.67 (1 in 149)	3.06 (1 in 33)	5.55 (1 in 18)
Lung/ Bronchus	0.03 (1 in 2,894)	0.94 (1 in 106)	3.98 (1 in 25)	5.69 (1 in 18)

SOURCE: American Cancer Society (www.cancer.org).

HOW BREAST CANCER GETS STARTED

How does cancer happen? It all starts with a single cell in the lining of the milk ducts. Every time a cell divides a small mistake can happen. Fortunately, mistakes only occur between 1 in 1 million and 1 in 100 million times.[38] Certain types of mistakes lead to cancer. A normal breast duct cell that divides begins to look and act like a breast duct. In other words, the cell differentiates. Cancer cells do not differentiate. They de-differentiate, meaning they look more embryonic and all the cells look alike.

The breast duct cell becomes odd looking and as it divides and multiplies, begins to fill the duct. This is called atypical hyperplasia. Most of the time this does not lead to cancer. But some of the time these atypical cells become even more bizarre looking. The more primitive the cell looks, the more deadly is the cancer. They fill the milk duct but do not go beyond it. This is called ductal carcinoma in situ or DCIS. DCIS can still technically be thought of as a precancer, because it has not broken out of the wall of the duct. If the cells do break through the wall of the duct into the fat around it—which it does 30% of the time— this is called invasion. If the cells invade deeper into the tissue and reach a blood vessel, they begin to spread to the rest of the body. This process, called metastasis, is what allows the cancer to be deadly.

If a woman's mother or sister has had the disease, especially before menopause, her risk of developing breast cancer increases. However, 70% to 80% of women who get the disease have no risk factors. Recently it has been discovered that some inherited genes can increase the risk of breast cancer. Two genes that have gotten a lot of attention are BRCA 1 (which is short for BReast CAncer 1) and BRCA 2 (which is short for BReast CAncer 2). The BRCA 1 gene is often found in families that have a lot of breast and ovarian cancer. The BRCA 2 gene is found more often in families that have a lot of male and female breast cancer. But 90% to 95% of those who develop breast cancer do not have either of these genes. So the first breast cancer cell, like those of other cancers, is more often caused by a combination of abnormal genes or substances in the environment or factors in a woman's life that can cause a normal gene or cell to mutate into cancer. That is one major reason why there is so much concern about estrogen and its possible link to breast cancer.

BREAST CANCER RISKS

- Age 65 or older
- Genetics—mother or sister with breast cancer, especially before menopause
- First period younger than age 12
- First child born after age 30
- Overweight more than 20%
- Excess alcohol—2 to 5 drinks daily increase risk by about 40%
- Lack of exercise—Exercising 3.8 hours a week can decrease your risk of breast cancer by 70% if you've had a child by age 30 and by 30% if you have not[39]
- Diet low in vegetables and fruit or high in fat
- Exposure to high-dose radiation
- Certain pesticides
- Long-term exposure to estrogen?

BREAST CANCER RISK AND ESTROGEN

A decade ago menopause was bad, estrogen was good, and life was easy. What could be bad? Breast cancer is what could be bad. Whether or not estrogen and/or progesterone increases the risk of breast cancer has emerged as one of the most important and challenging questions facing women as they enter menopause. It also challenges doctors as they try to offer advice on risk versus benefit of hormone replacement therapy (HRT) to their patients. We know that estrogen will treat hot flashes, help prevent osteoporosis, and lower LDL, or bad cholesterol, and may prevent heart disease in healthy women. It may also prevent or delay Alzheimer's disease. We'll talk a lot more about this in Chapter 2. But the controversy is: Does estrogen increase the risk of breast cancer?

Studies offer conflicting results. This is particularly true for women who have used estrogen for 5 to 15 years in whom some studies suggest a 30% to 40% increased risk of breast cancer. First, it is important to understand exactly what this does not mean. It does not mean that there is a 30% to 40% risk of breast cancer if you use estrogen for a long time. The important word here is *increased*. For instance, if the risk of breast cancer without taking estrogen is 10 per 100 by age 80, the risk after 5 to 15 years of taking estrogen would be 13 to 14 per 100 (30% to 40% more than 10). Does that mean that if you ever popped an estrogen tablet into your mouth your risk for breast cancer might be a tad greater? No! Almost every study shows that taking estrogen for 5 years or less does not increase the risk of breast cancer. But there is a cloud surrounding estrogen, which is one of the reasons women are seeking alternatives such as soy.

Ovarian Cancer

Newsweek magazine asked, "What did comedienne Gilda Radner, singer Laura Nyro, and actress Jessica Tandy have in common?" The answer was "All three were great performers—and all three died of ovarian cancer."[40] Although it is much less common than breast cancer (1 in 57 versus 1 in 8 over a lifetime) it is much more deadly. Of the 23,100 women diagnosed in 2000, almost 14,000 will die.[41] Why so many? Because two thirds of the time it has spread widely (stage III) before it is diagnosed. By then the cure rate is a disappointing 20%. If it is found early, which occurs in only 25% of cases, the cure rate is excellent.

One of my patients, Debby, came to me in her early 30s hoping to start her family. She had no symptoms at all. While investigating her infertility I found a cyst on her ovary that turned out to be early ovarian cancer. She was treated, cured, and later went on to conceive. Had this cancer not been found, she might have been treated with fertility drugs and thought that they caused her cancer, or worse yet, she might have died.

Why is ovarian cancer so hard to diagnose? First of all the symptoms are vague—mild abdominal bloating, fullness after eating small amounts, constipation, indigestion, and frequent urination. Second, tests like the Pap smear do not pick it up and blood tests like CA-125 are often falsely positive or negative. I have screened patients with CA-125 whose levels were quite elevated only to find the levels returning to normal after removing a breast cyst, endometriosis from their pelvic organs, or a fibroid tumor from their uterus. In the meantime, they were worried sick that they had ovarian cancer. I think the CA-125 causes more worry than it provides help.

What is a good test? An ultrasound of the ovaries. I believe every woman after age 50 should have one every 2 years along with an annual pelvic exam. Insurance often will not pay for the ultrasound because they say it is not cost effective. Translation: It is cheaper for them to pay for the 23,100 women who get ovarian cancer than to pay for the millions of ultrasounds that would be negative. Women who have had a pregnancy, who breast-fed, or who used oral contraceptives (5 years of use cuts your risk in half) are at lower risk for ovarian cancer. If you have never been pregnant, have a family history of breast or ovarian cancer, or have a high-fat diet, your risk increases. If you are in this category, get the ultrasound, even if you have to pay for it.

Endometrial (Uterine) Cancer

The lining of the uterus is called the endometrium, so cancers that begin in the glands that line the uterus are called endometrial cancer. According to the North American Menopause Society, fewer than 3 in 100 women at age 50 will develop this cancer in their remaining life. Still that translates into 36,100 new cases in 2000 of which 6,500 will die.

RISK FACTORS FOR UTERINE CANCER

- Obesity
- Diabetes
- High blood pressure
- Gallbladder disease
- Absent or very infrequent periods before menopause
- Using estrogen (especially higher dosages) without progesterone—using progesterone with estrogen virtually eliminates this risk
- Prolonged use of tamoxifen?

This disease is most common between the ages of 55 and 70, and the most common symptom is abnormal uterine bleeding (bleeding that occurs at a time other than when it is expected, if you are still menstruating or taking birth control pills or estrogen and/or progesterone, or any time at all if you are already in menopause). If you are about to begin estrogen replacement, get an endometrial biopsy first. Soy protects the uterine lining and does not stimulate it to grow.

Cervical Cancer

Cervical cancer is the disease that is tested for by the Pap smear—a test introduced in the 1930s. If all women had this test done each year, the risk of dying from cervical cancer would approach zero. That is why the risk of dying from this disease has dropped by 75% since 1940. Unfortunately, there will be 12,900 new diagnoses of cervical cancer in 2001 and 4,400 deaths. Get a Pap smear and stop worrying about this cancer.[42]

RISK FACTORS FOR CERVICAL CANCER

- Sexual intercourse at an early age
- Multiple male sexual partners
- Male sexual partners who have had multiple partners
- HIV-positive status
- Smoking

Colon and Rectal Cancer

The colon is the lower part of the intestine and the rectum is the final segment that leads from the colon to the anus. This cancer is still very common in American women (68,600 new cases and 28,800 deaths in 2000) and like many cancers, it is more likely to occur between the time that menopause begins and age 75. The good news is that this year, rates of colon and rectal cancer among women are beginning to decline. Your risk of getting this type of cancer may be reduced by exercising, eating healthfully, and possibly by estrogen replacement therapy. Soy may also lower your risk for colon cancer (see Chapter 7). Other factors can increase your risk for this disease. They include:

RISK FACTORS FOR COLON AND RECTAL CANCER

- Family history of this disease
- Colorectal polyps

- Inflammatory bowel disease
- Lack of exercise?
- High-fat, low-fiber diet?

Like many cancers, the most common symptom is abnormal bleeding. Any bleeding from the rectum, especially after menopause, should cause you to call your doctor and find out why. You can also screen for colon and rectal cancer. Each year after 40 and definitely after age 50, have a rectal exam and have the stool tested for blood. This simple test is usually done in your doctor's office and the results are given to you during the exam. After age 50, it is also advisable to have a flexible sigmoidoscopy (view inside the rectum and lower colon) every 3 to 5 years to check for any cancer or precancerous growths. If the cancer is found before it has spread, 91% of those treated will survive five years or more.

chapter 2

HORMONE REPLACEMENT THERAPY: EVALUATING THE RISKS AND BENEFITS

HOW MANY WOMEN TAKE HORMONE REPLACEMENT THERAPY?

Premarin, the number one selling medication in the United States, has annual sales of more than $5 billion. Sounds like everyone must be using it. But that is not the case. The reality is that only about 15% to 20% of postmenopausal women in the United States use estrogen for more than 1 year.

How does this stack up to women in other parts of the world? It is much the same percentages overall in Europe, although it varies from country to country. For instance, in Italy and Spain it's about 3%; in Denmark and in the Netherlands, about 12%; and in Germany, 20% to 25%. In France and England it is slightly less than in Germany and rather similar to the percentage seen in the United States.[1]

These differences may reflect the enthusiasm that doctors have for recommending estrogen. Consider a report from South Australia where the rate of postmenopausal estrogen use doubled from 1991 to 1995—not only the rate of new users but also the number of women who used it for 5 years or longer. How did the Australians do it? Through an enormous educational effort for both the medical profession and the public.[2] Make no mistake, how well and how enthusiastically doctors and the rest of the medical community understand and explain the risks and benefits of estrogen therapy has an enormous impact on how many postmenopausal women use it and for how long.

BUT IS IT SAFE?

The subject of estrogen causes lively discussion. Doctors and talk show hosts, journalists and patients all are willing to oblige. Some love it, and some hate it. But just about everyone has a strong opinion. It is because over the past few decades, hormone replacement therapy (HRT), and estrogen in particular, has gone through a revolution and a counterrevolution. This should not be surprising because the hormone in question has the potential to do a lot of good and, according to a growing number of studies, the potential to do a lot of harm.

I will not try to persuade you that estrogen is either good or bad, because it can be both. It depends on you as an individual—your age, your weight, your medical history, what other medications you are taking, which progesterone you use, and whether or not you smoke—whether it is right for you or not. It is a decision you can make only after discussing your medical history and the risks and benefits of estrogen with your doctor.

In this chapter, I will talk about the effect of the body's estrogen on the breasts at different ages, a brief history of estrogen as a medication, and the risks and benefits of taking it. I will also describe the major studies on estrogen replacement therapy and discuss what they tell us and why they confuse us. The difficulty is not lack of information, but the enormous and growing amount of information that has to be assimilated and individualized.

HOW THE BODY'S ESTROGEN AFFECTS THE BREASTS AT DIFFERENT AGES

Throughout a woman's life, the estrogen produced naturally by her body has an effect on her breasts. Early in puberty, when estrogen is just starting to be produced but before ovulation and progesterone production begins, the ducts of the breasts begin to increase and branch (see Figure 2-1). Later in puberty, ovulation begins and with it, the production of progesterone, which stimulates the alveolar cells to start developing. Without progesterone, these changes do not occur. When a girl enters her reproductive years, she develops regular menstrual cycles, causing the tips (called the terminal end buds) of the breast ducts, but not the bases, to divide more rapidly. From this time until menopause, the breasts are in a constant state of change with each menstrual cycle—denser in the first half than in the second.[3]

After menopause, estrogen and progesterone levels are lower, and there is less cell division in the breasts. Both the ducts and the alveolar tissue become quiet and the breasts

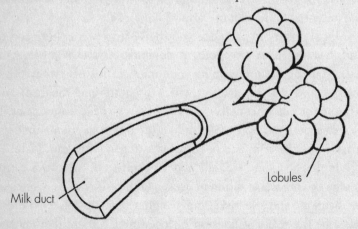

Lobules

Milk duct

FIGURE 2-1.   Microanatomy of Breast
SOURCE: Modified from Love S, Lindsey K. *Dr. Susan Love's Hormone Book*. New York: Random House; 1997.

become smaller as the tips of the ducts but not the base shrink in size. However, the cells of the breast remember estrogen and progesterone, and if they are exposed to these hormones later in life, they quickly respond and enlarge again.

A major consequence of menopause on the breasts is that fat replaces the denser tissue. These changes allow mammograms to see into the breasts of postmenopausal women not on HRT much more easily than into the breasts of premenopausal women.[4] As you have probably already guessed, HRT stimulates the already sensitized breast tissue to become denser, fuller, and larger.[5] This increased density may include the entire breast, several small areas, or one specific area. Benign breast masses, including fibroadenomas and cysts (so-called fibrocystic disease or lumpy breasts), become more common.[6] All of these changes make mammograms a little more difficult for the radiologist to read and sometimes trigger additional mammograms, ultrasounds, and even biopsies to be performed. Once HRT is discontinued, the radiologist's ability to read a mammogram is the same as for women who have never used HRT.[7]

Selective estrogen receptor modulators, or so-called SERMs, are estrogen-like hormones that have been modified to act like estrogen on the bones and like an antiestrogen on the breasts. Two examples are raloxifene (which is typically used to treat osteoporosis) and tamoxifen (which is typically used to treat breast cancer). Once we realize that estrogen and progesterone are supposed to have an effect on breast tissue and that the specific effects change at different points of the life cycle, it is easy to understand how scientific studies on the effect of HRT on the breasts can become confusing.

In 1966 Robert A. Wilson, M.D., wrote a book called *Feminine Forever*.[8] It was a turning point for estrogen, which at that time was a relatively new drug with a lot of potential. By potential I mean the preliminary information looked promising and it could be mass produced and made available at a reasonable cost.

TABLE 2-1. A BRIEF HISTORY OF ESTROGEN

1912	Ovarian extracts injected into virgin animals causes estrus
1913	First ovarian extract
1923	Estrogen first synthesized
1938	Diethylstilbestrol (DES) is mass produced, making it both plentiful and cheap
1941	Estrogen first approved for human use
1942	Conjugated equine estrogen (CEE) such as Premarin approved for menopause
1966	Dr. Robert A. Wilson writes *Feminine Forever* and glorifies the benefits of estrogen
2000	National Toxicology Program Advisory Committee recommends that estrogens be listed as "known to be human carcinogen." Risks versus benefits of estrogen in question
2002	WHI study discontinued due to breast cancer risks. NCI study warns of estrogen causing ovarian cancer

At the same time, women were hoping not to suffer with the symptoms of menopause and were looking for an option to help them stay symptom free, healthy, and more youthful.

Enter Dr. Wilson, who wrote in his book that it was "unnecessary for women to suffer in a civilized world." His basic premise was that a woman in menopause has lower levels of estrogen, and if she would take estrogen she could retain her beauty, her sexuality, and her youth for an extended period of time. The message was simple, the meaning was clear. After menopause, estrogen levels become lower and women get older and suffer more ills. He reasoned that as women reached menopause they should embrace estrogen. Estrogen was good, its effects were good. End of discussion!

Armed with a firm belief in its virtues, estrogen replacement became a sermon preached to the masses by enthusiastic doctors who now had an antidote for the natural consequences of aging. Every woman who was approaching or in menopause was encouraged to drink from the fountain of youth. The argument was simple and compelling, and the timing was right. It is easy to understand the zeal of the medical community and the willingness of the masses to be converted.

The enormous and widespread use of estrogen set the stage for today's confusion. Just about everybody was given estrogen. It was prescribed to women without considering the risks to a specific individual. An extreme example happened in the mid-1960s. Estrogen was believed to be so beneficial for reducing the risk of heart disease that it was even prescribed to men with a history of heart disease. The results were disastrous—instead of reducing the risk of heart disease in men, high-dose estrogen caused more nonfatal heart attacks, pulmonary emboli, and deaths than a placebo. Today we know a lot more about the importance of the individual medical history. Prescribing selectively is the only way to maximize the benefits and minimize the risks of taking estrogen.

FIRST, THE BENEFITS

This may sound obvious, but one of the best ways to determine if you will benefit from HRT is to have a clear reason for taking it. The fact that you are approaching menopause or are in menopause is not a reason by itself. Estrogen has the potential to affect your entire body, from the organs and blood vessels within you to the skin that surrounds you. For that reason, ask yourself what it is you want from taking estrogen. Are you bothered by hot flashes? Do you think you are at risk for developing osteoporosis? Are you having a problem with loss of urine? Is there a family history of heart disease or Alzheimer's disease?

A clear question is the best way to get a clear answer to "Is HRT right for me?" Specific questions can be discussed with your doctor in the form of risks and benefits to you from HRT. Other treatment options available to treat your problem should be examined. You are much more likely to get the information you need with this approach.

Hot Flashes

If hot flashes are your biggest problem, estrogen will solve it for you about 95% of the time.[9] That is why the Food and Drug Administration (FDA) approved estrogen for the treatment of hot flashes. It may not happen overnight (about 40% of women will experience an immediate effect), but within a few weeks you will start to notice a difference. By 4 weeks the majority of women will experience relief. Reducing the number of hot flashes may have another beneficial effect. Women who have less hot flashes also have less sleep disturbances. Once you have been able to sleep undisturbed, you may find that both your memory and your mood are positively affected.

If you are planning to start taking estrogen because you are premenopausal and scheduled for surgery to remove your ovaries, start taking the estrogen within 1 or 2 days following the procedure. After that, any estrogen still in your bloodstream will have passed out of your body and very strong hot flashes will begin.

If you have been taking estrogen for a while and want to

quit, do not stop taking it all at once or your symptoms probably will return. Wean your body off the medication gradually. There are a number of ways to do this, and you should discuss these with your doctor. You can try taking one less pill each week for a month at a time until you are down to only one pill a week before going cold turkey. If you are using an estrogen patch, remove the patch a day earlier each week for a month, then 2 days earlier for the next month, and so on. If you are using progesterone along with the estrogen, keep using the usual dosage until you have weaned yourself completely off the estrogen. Sometimes, even doing it this way, the hot flashes return. One bit of good news along these lines: If you did not have hot flashes before starting estrogen, you probably will not have them when you come off.[10]

What if you do not want to take estrogen? Progesterone has been shown to lower hot flashes in 70% of patients using it. However, progesterone has been credited with causing some of the more unpleasant side effects associated with taking hormone replacement therapy, such as water retention, irritability, mood swings, waking up groggy, and having breast tenderness. Synthetic progestins, such as medroxyprogesterone acetate, are more likely to cause these problems than natural progesterone. One approach you may want to discuss with your physician is using 1 gram (one-quarter teaspoon) of 3% strength natural progesterone cream or gels, applied twice daily, either directly to the breasts, the lower abdomen, or the inner thighs. You can increase the potency to 6%, and even to 10%, should it be needed. Pro-Gest is a nonprescription natural progesterone cream that is available in 1.5% strength. Capsules of natural progesterone are also available at 25 milligrams (mg) taken 3 times daily. These doses can be slowly increased to 50, 75, and even 100 mg. Once you are able to sleep through the night, your dosage is correct. If you experience any of the side effects of progesterone that I mentioned above, cut back a little until you find the optimum dosage for you.

If you have not had a hysterectomy (your uterus removed), unless you are taking a very low dose of estrogen, you will have to take progesterone along with the estrogen for at least 10 days of each month to protect the uterine lining from developing precancerous changes. In addition to the progesterone options that I mentioned, a vaginal cream called Crinone that comes in 4% and 8% strengths is also available.

Osteoporosis

Most of the calcium our bones will ever have, 91% of it, will get there by age 17.[11] In the years that follow, we simply try to stop our bones from losing what we stored up to that time. From age 35 until menopause, bone loss speeds up to a rate of 1% per year. After menopause, the rate of bone loss increases even more, to 3% per year for the first 5 years and then slows down to 1% per year.

For more than a quarter of a century, it has been known that estrogen replacement helps prevent osteoporosis.[12] However, once bone is lost, estrogen generally does not put much bone back. A classic study showed that when estrogen was given to premenopausal women shortly after surgery to remove their ovaries, they did not develop osteoporosis. If they waited 3 to 6 years after surgery to start taking estrogen, they did lose some bone density. Once they started taking the estrogen they did not lose any more bone. A study published in 2000 added a little fine tuning to this point.[13] After 3 years of taking at least 80% of their estrogen pills, either alone or with progesterone, only 8% of women had lost bone in their spines, compared to 40% of women who took a placebo. HRT also prevented bone loss from hip measurements—11.8% of women taking HRT lost bone compared with 35.4% of women not taking HRT. The study also pointed out that approximately half of untreated women do not lose bone after menopause.

In summary, get a bone-density test before you start taking estrogen and another one a year or so later, whether or not you take estrogen to prevent osteoporosis. It is the only way to be certain if you need to start treatment for osteoporosis or if the estrogen is working.

Just about every estrogen fights osteoporosis. It doesn't seem to matter whether you are taking a conjugated equine estrogen (CEE) such as Premarin in dosages of 0.625 mg per day[14] or 0.3 mg per day,[15] a dose of 0.5 mg per day of oral estradiol, or an estradiol patch in dosages as low as 0.025 mg per day,[16] although a slightly higher dose of 0.05 mg per day works a little better.[17] The lower dose of the patch works because the estrogen in it is absorbed through the skin rather than through the intestinal tract where it is broken down in the liver causing a large portion of it to be lost.

Overall, the use of estrogen (and probably other drugs that are used to treat osteoporosis) reduces the risk of breaking your hip by about 50%.[18] But taking estrogen does not guarantee it will never happen. An 80-year-old woman who has taken estrogen since menopause will lose only 10% of her bone density, compared to the 30% lost by a woman of the same age who has never taken estrogen.[19] For that reason, even if you are taking estrogen you still need to get a bone-density test.

Breaking your hip is not the only risk of having osteoporosis. Losing bone will also increase the chances of losing your teeth because the maxilla and mandible (that is, your jaw bone) provides the framework for tooth support. Estrogen can help prevent that from happening[20] and may even play a role in reducing the risk of gingival inflammation and progression to periodontitis in women with osteoporosis who are early in menopause.[21] Other common bone problems due to osteoporosis include compression of the backbone causing loss of height and a "dowager's hump," and fractures of the wrist and forearm.

One last point about estrogen and osteoporosis. Do not forget to take your calcium and vitamin D along with it.[22] Taking calcium along with estrogen does a better job of preventing osteoporosis than either estrogen or calcium alone—particularly if you are taking low doses of estrogen.[23] If you are taking a magnesium supplement as well, it is best to take it at a different time than the calcium and not in combination. Magnesium and calcium compete with each other for absorption into the body, and taking both together may actually allow slightly less of each into the bloodstream. I'll talk more about the differences between calcium supplements in Chapter 5.

Loss of Urine

Half of all menopausal women will have at least some urine loss that is severe enough to cause a social or hygienic problem and 25% will need surgery to correct it. According to a 1995 report in the *Lancet,* the direct health-care costs related to loss of urine in 1987 were a staggering $10 billion, which is greater than the cost of dialysis and coronary artery bypass surgery combined.[24] That is because the urethra—the tube that carries urine from the bladder out of the body—is much shorter in women than it is in men. Also the wear and tear of childbirth can weaken the pelvic muscles and the fascia, which is the fibrous sheath that reinforces and additionally supports the urethra.[25] This is why women who have had children are more likely to have urine loss than those who have not. However, even among female varsity athletes who have never had children, 28% experience some episodes of urine loss during sports participation.[26] The lining of the urethra and the fascia and the pelvic muscles that surround them all are sensitive to estrogen, and all often weaken in menopause as estrogen levels decline. Less pelvic support allows a cough or sneeze to force out urine. (See Chapter 1, Urinary Tract Problems.)

Lower estrogen levels also change the type of bacteria that normally live in the vagina.[27] During the reproductive years, the

TABLE 2-2. COMMON GENITOURINARY SYMPTOMS ASSOCIATED WITH REDUCED ESTROGEN

Irritation	Frequent urination
Burning	Urgent need to urinate
Itching	Painful urination
Discharge	Waking up at night to urinate
Painful intercourse	Loss of urine (incontinence)
Shortening/narrowing of the vagina	

predominant bacteria in the vagina are lactobacilli. After menopause, estrogen levels decrease, which causes the acidity, or pH, of the vagina to increase. That allows new types of bacteria, including some that can cause bladder infections, to survive in the vagina and infect the nearby bladder.

Estrogen increases blood flow to the pelvis, adding strength to the tissues and support to the bladder. It also lowers the pH, which together with the increased blood flow makes the vagina more resistant to vaginitis or inflammation called atrophic vaginitis. Estrogen placed in the vagina within rings that look something like a diaphragm has been shown to also reduce the risk of a urinary tract infection.[28-30]

Mood and Thought

One benefit of estrogen that may be increasingly important is its effect on mood and thought. There is a large and growing amount of research showing that estrogen has a very positive effect on the brain. It may help prevent memory loss, maintain a better quality of life, and have a positive influence on mood. There is also very strong evidence that estrogen might help stave off the development of Alzheimer's disease, although it does not appear to be able to help treat it.[31-36] Estrogen's effect on the brain may prove to be one of its most important potential benefits.

Other Potential Benefits of Estrogen

In addition to the benefits listed above, a few others should at least be mentioned. Women who suffer menstrual migraines may find that using estrogen reduces their frequency in the perimenopause.[37] Best results seem to occur using a natural estrogen combination such as Tri-Est gel, ½ to 1½ grams, 2 to 3 times daily beginning 1 to 2 days before the expected headache and continuing through the menstrual period. Estrogen may also lower the risk for macular degeneration, a condition that can lead to visual loss primarily after the age of 60[38] and may also lower the risk of colon cancer.[39] Estrogen also plays an important role in preventing collagen loss. Collagen is a substance that is important for both bone and skin. Thirty percent of skin collagen is lost in the first 5 years after menopause. This is part of the explanation for estrogen's beneficial effect on osteoporosis and urine leakage, and also partially explains why skin wrinkles and ages faster after menopause. It is also how estrogen helps that problem. To protect your skin from wrinkles, start taking estrogen soon after menopause to prevent the fall-off in collagen.

THE RISKS OF HRT

Two of the most common worries about using HRT are abnormal uterine bleeding and fear of developing breast cancer. Every medication comes with potential risks, and HRT is no exception. As you will see, some of the risks are idiosyncratic, meaning there is no good way to tell who is more likely to experience them. But others are much more likely to occur in certain individuals (see Risk Factors for Taking Estrogen). If you are at higher risk, think twice before taking estrogen. Every medical decision involves weighing the risks and the benefits. You should already know why you want to take estrogen. Discuss HRT with your doctor. Be sure that in your case, the benefits of HRT out-weigh the risks. If they do not, consider alternative choices such as soy.

Risk Factors for Taking Estrogen

- History of blood clots or stroke
- History of heart disease
- History of breast or uterine cancer
- Liver disease
- Gallbladder disease
- Irregular bleeding of unknown cause
- Smoking

Endometrial (Uterine) Cancer

Estrogen can cause the cells of the uterine lining to go through changes that lead to cancer. The risk is about 2 to 8 times greater than for the general population.[40] Fortunately, the risk of precan-cerous changes (called hyperplasia) is greater than the risk of cancer per se. The chance of hyperplasia occurring may be as high as 20% in just 1 year and 40% in 3 years.[41] While this sounds pretty bleak, the good news is that only 1% to 3% of these is thought to progress to uterine cancer if left untreated.

There is very good news about preventing estrogen from causing uterine cancer. Today, uterine cancer caused by estrogen is rapidly becoming a thing of the past. The reason is simple. Giving progesterone along with estrogen for at least 10 days of the month almost completely eliminates the risk of uterine can-cer. Unfortunately, the key word is almost. In some rare cases, uterine cancer still occurs even if you take both estrogen and progesterone.[42] If you are taking estrogen and if you still have your uterus, I recommend being checked each year or two for uterine cancer.

It is relatively easy to detect an abnormal uterine lining before it has time to become cancerous. The uterine lining should be checked before you start taking estrogen and once a year after that. The two main ways of checking the uterine lining are by endometrial biopsy and a transvaginal ultrasound. Both are office procedures. For the endometrial biopsy, a small catheter is inserted into the uterus. A few cells are removed and looked at under a microscope. This procedure causes some cramps but only lasts a few minutes. Local anesthesia and/or a mild pain reliever can make the biopsy more comfortable. A transvaginal ultrasound is done by placing a probe about the width of your thumb into your vagina and measuring the thickness of the uterine lining. It is painless, can be done with an empty bladder, and only takes a few minutes. If the uterine lining is 4 millimeters (mm) or less, you can relax. If the lining is more than 4 mm your doctor may want to do the endometrial biopsy also.

Ovarian Cancer

Most studies on estrogen replacement therapy did not raise a red flag about estrogen increasing the risk of ovarian cancer. But that changed with an article published in March 2001.[43] A group of 211,581 postmenopausal women with no history of cancer, hysterectomy, or surgery on their ovaries were followed from 1982 until 1996. Women who took estrogen for more than 10 years were more likely to die of ovarian cancer than women who had never taken estrogen. However, the risk decreased each year after the estrogen was stopped. Overall, when all the women who had ever used estrogen were considered together, regardless of how long they took it or when they quit, the average risk of dying from ovarian cancer was 1.23 times that of those women who never used it. A similar study from NCI in July 2002, found comparable results. These studies reinforce my belief that postmenopausal women, especially those who take estrogen, should have a pelvic ultrasound at least every 2 years in addition to their annual pelvic exams.

Blood Clots

Several studies have observed that taking estrogen slightly increases the risk of blood clots (venous thrombosis), especially in the first year of taking it.[44-46] If a blood clot is going to happen, it does not seem to matter what estrogen dose a person is taking. But we learned from the July 2002 Women's Health Initiative study the risk may increase if they are taking medroxyprogesterone. Fortunately, the blood clots are rarely fatal and the actual risk small.[47] If you have a history of blood clots, especially if you smoke, estrogen will likely put you at increased risk of having another.

To give the risk of using estrogen some perspective, compare it with what happens without taking estrogen. The overall risk of a blood clot without taking estrogen is 11/100,000 women. If the risk more than doubled to 25/100,000 women, that would still be less than half of the 60/100,000 women who get blood clots during normal pregnancies. If you have a history of blood clots or migraine headaches, do not take estrogen without a long and clear discussion with your doctor. If you do not have a history of blood clots but are still worried about the risk, ask your doctor to test your blood to measure your coagulation factors. Those measurements will tell if your blood clots normally or faster than it should. If your blood clots too fast do not take estrogen. Another type of blood test will measure a protein called homocysteine. Homocysteine occurs normally in the body as part of metabolism. If the level of homocysteine is too high, it can lead to hardening of the arteries (atherosclerosis) and blood clots. If your homocysteine levels are elevated, discuss taking folic acid, B_6, and B_{12} with your doctor. Often these vitamins will lower the elevated homocysteine levels into the normal range so that taking estrogen does not create a problem.

High Blood Pressure

High blood pressure (hypertension) happens in about 5% of women who take birth control pills. But, for the overwhelming percentage of women, estrogen has either no effect on blood pressure or may actually reduce it. If you begin taking estrogen and notice an increase in either your systolic (the top number) or diastolic (the bottom number), simply stopping the estrogen will reverse the problem. Sometimes changing the dosage or how you take the estrogen will also do the trick.

RISK AND BENEFIT CONTROVERSIES

Estrogen has been in the news so much recently that people are really getting confused and worried about two very important questions:

- Is estrogen good for your heart?
- Is estrogen bad for your breasts?

These are good questions, and the answers help explain why women should or should not choose estrogen. Gallup polls show that most women believe they will die of breast cancer when, in fact, they are 10 times more likely to die of heart disease (see Table 2-3).[48] The absolute chance of dying of breast cancer between the ages of 50 and 70 is 4.7%, and the risk of dying of it in that same 20-year period is 1.04%.[49]

Therefore, if estrogen is good for your cardiovascular system it could play a major beneficial role in your overall health. If estrogen increases your risk of developing breast cancer, it is ter-

TABLE 2-3. WOMEN'S TOP HEALTH CONCERNS AND ACTUAL CAUSES OF DEATH

Perception	(%)	Actual Risk	(%)
Breast cancer	46	Breast cancer	4
Cancer in general	16	Other cancers	12
Heart disease	4	Heart disease	34
AIDS	4	Lung cancer	5
Uterus/ovarian cancer	3	Stroke	8

SOURCE: Gallup poll.

rible. Also, it feeds into the very health concern that troubles women most—that they will die of breast cancer.

Historically, estrogen was thought to be good for the heart and its effect on the breasts was neutral. Today, some new data suggests that estrogen is neutral for the heart and bad for the breasts. It is not that simple. It comes down to benefit, risk, and you as an individual. I will not say that estrogen is either universally good or bad for hearts and breasts. Look at the following information. It might help you make a better decision for yourself.

HRT and Breast Cancer—Controversy and Anxiety

ESTROGEN HISTORY THAT INCREASES BREAST CANCER RISK

- Early menarche—the earlier your first period, the more cycles of estrogen production
- Late first full-term pregnancy
- Late menopause—the later your last period, the more cycles of estrogen production

There are many kinds of HRT. In the United States most studies have been done with the conjugated equine estrogen Premarin and the synthetic progesterone Provera. In contrast, most of the reports on HRT that come from Europe were done with oral 17-beta estradiol. Also, taking estrogen plus progesterone is known to lower the risk of uterine cancer, but it could be riskier for breast cancer than taking estrogen alone. Finally, breast cancer risk with HRT might be greater if you are thin than if you are overweight. A possible explanation for this is that fat cells manufacture estrogen. Thin people produce relatively lower estrogen levels and are at lower risk of getting breast cancer until they take HRT.

These last two points come up in several articles, but they are not agreed upon by everyone.

Early in 2000, the National Cancer Institute (NCI) reported their findings on the risk of breast cancer facing post-menopausal women who chose to take either estrogen alone or estrogen combined with progesterone.[50] Their findings generated a lot of excitement. Women who were taking HRT or had taken it within 4 years of being diagnosed with breast cancer were more likely to get the disease if they took both estrogen and progesterone than if they were taking estrogen alone. This report and another[51] found there was an increased risk of breast cancer among women who used estrogen alone only in those women who were both thin and used estrogen for 6 years or more. Women who took both estrogen and progesterone were also more likely to develop breast cancer if they were thin.

Another study[52] also found an increased risk of breast cancer among women who took estrogen plus progesterone compared with estrogen alone, but this difference was not statistically significant. The National Cancer Institute also reported that taking estrogen and progesterone sequentially (taking estrogen all month and progesterone only part of the month) was riskier than taking both hormones daily in combination. However, the women who took only estrogen did not have an increased risk of developing breast cancer even if they took it for 15 years or more.

There are at least three studies that show estrogen used with progesterone increases the risk of breast cancer[53-55] but nine others do *not* show a significant increase.[56-64]

There is also disagreement whether obese postmenopausal women are at more or less risk of breast cancer than their thin counterparts. Here is why. As I explained earlier, obese women make more estrogen in their fat cells than thin women. This extra estrogen causes another hormone called sex hormone binding globulin (SHBG) to be reduced. Why does this matter? Because SHBG "binds" almost all the estrogen in the bloodstream, leaving only the "unbound" or "free" estrogen to be active in the body. The less SHBG, the more free estrogen to affect the breast.[65] Several studies have shown that post-menopausal women who have higher blood levels of free estradiol are more likely to develop breast cancer.[66] However, at the same time, obese premenopausal women tend to have longer menstrual cycles and fewer ovulations each year than non-obese premenopausal women do, and less ovulations cause less exposure to estrogen and a reduced risk of breast cancer.[67]

Clearly, there is no consensus. These seemingly contradictory facts are enough to confuse anyone—and confusion is the source of all the anxiety. The bottom line is that everyone agrees that taking estrogen for 5 years or less should have little effect on your risk for breast cancer. Unfortunately, for the immediate future, whether or not taking estrogen alone for 5 to 10 years or more increases your risk of breast cancer cannot be answered. The July 2002 Women's Health Initiative study (JAMA), strongly suggests that taking estrogen with medroxyprogesterone (but not necessarily other progesterones) does slightly increase the risk of breast cancer. A separate WHI study looking at the risks of estrogen alone is still ongoing. There is one very positive note in all of this. If you have been on estrogen in the past and your fear of future breast cancer is driving you crazy, do not despair. Whatever the risk, as soon as you come off HRT your risk starts to come down. After being off the hormones for 5 years, any increased risk of breast cancer due to taking HRT seems to be removed.[68]

BREAST CANCER SURVIVAL IN POSTMENOPAUSAL HORMONE USERS

There is something positive for women who have taken HRT and get breast cancer. Their cancer is usually at an earlier stage (less likely to have spread) and less aggressive, and they usually have a much better chance of surviving than women who get breast cancer and have not taken HRT.[69–72] These biologic differences imply that hormone treatment promotes the growth of a malignant cluster of cells already in place rather than turning normal tissue into cancer.[73] As you might expect, not everyone agrees with this view either.

Another encouraging point comes from the Breast Cancer Detection Project, designed to screen women for breast cancer. In that study, women who were currently taking HRT when they were diagnosed with breast cancer had a 40% to 60% better chance of surviving up to 12 years after their diagnosis than those women not taking HRT.[74] Once again, this points to a better survival among women who take HRT and unfortunately develop breast cancer than among women who have not.

All of this creates very complicated questions for the nearly 2.5 million breast cancer survivors in the United States today. Breast cancer is being discovered sooner at both an earlier age and an earlier stage than in the past, and many of those women are treated with chemotherapy that often destroys their ovaries and makes them menopausal. Of course, the earlier the stage of breast cancer, the more likely will be the cure. Should these women consider HRT to treat their symptoms?

Before you decide this is a completely far-fetched notion,

let me tell you that there are an increasing number of prospective studies that show women with localized breast cancer who later took HRT do not have an increased rate of recurrence over similar women who do not take estrogen.[75] I will discuss this further in Chapter 7. This is a situation that clearly comes with some risk. In many cases it is safer to consider alternatives to estrogen for treating the symptoms of menopause (see Chapter 9). Clearly, if you do want to use estrogen in this situation, work closely with your doctor, know what symptoms you want to treat, and what your alternatives are. If you still want to use HRT, use the lowest dosage possible.[76]

PROGESTERONE AND THE BREAST

Is estrogen plus progesterone a greater risk for breast cancer than estrogen alone? This question is important and the answer is confusing. We do know that women who still have their uterus and take estrogen typically also need progesterone to protect their uterine lining from developing precancerous changes. But is progesterone's effect on the breast different than its effect on the uterus?

There are studies showing that breast tissue is more actively dividing in the second half of the menstrual cycle when progesterone levels are naturally highest.[77] Some scientists think this increased cell division leads to genetic "mistakes" that later develop into breast cancer.[78] Other studies use this information to recommend that breast cancer surgery be performed in the first half of the menstrual cycle when progesterone levels are lowest to improve outcome if cancer is found.

Two large clinical studies caused a great deal of concern. One report from the University of Southern California, February 2000, compared hormone use in 1,897 postmenopausal women diagnosed with breast cancer and 1,637 similarly matched post-menopausal women who did not have the disease. Breast cancer risk rose 24% for every 5 years of use among women using combined estrogen and progesterone, compared to an increased risk of 6% (an amount not considered statistically significant) if the patients were on estrogen only.[79] The other report, published in January 2000, used information from a National Cancer Institute breast screening program. The researchers found that women taking a combined estrogen and progesterone regimen increased their risk of breast cancer by 8% for each year they took combined HRT compared with 1% per year on estrogen alone.[80]

Unfortunately, both of these studies were flawed, and these flaws caused the reliability of the findings to fall short of actually proving a relationship between breast cancer risk and HRT. Both studies used information about HRT that came from recollection. Study designers agree that people who depend on recall to answer questions are more likely to answer either inaccurately or in a biased way. The *JAMA* study also fell short because the number of women taking estrogen and progesterone was quite small compared with the number taking estrogen only. Other flaws have also been cited that might have skewed the conclusions.

But not all information points to a negative effect of progesterone. Progesterone levels are not higher in women who ultimately develop breast cancer.[81] And human breast tissue specimens removed from patients treated with estrogen and progesterone indicate that progesterone slows down estrogen's stimulating effect on the breast.[82] Even when human breast cancer cells are treated with progesterone in petri dishes, breast cancer cell growth slows down.[83]

It will take more time and study to find answers to this question. At the present time, it seems that progesterone may add a slight additional risk to the development of breast cancer. Avoiding the synthetic progesterone medroxyprogesterone acetate may reduce this potential increase in risk.

HRT and the Risk of Heart Disease

Diseases of the heart and blood vessels (cardiovascular disease) are the most common cause of death among postmenopausal women. In 1997, cardiovascular disease killed one-half million American women, more than the next 14 causes of death combined.[84] Because the number is so large, even a small reduction in the number of deaths is important.

Believe it or not, even though there is an enormous amount of discussion about HRT and heart disease and the benefits it may provide, there are no large, published, randomized studies that show HRT protects the heart. However, a number of epidemiological studies have suggested that HRT reduces the risk of dying from cardiovascular disease by 40% to 50% in healthy users.[85] In other words, in women who do not already have heart disease. A great deal of additional research supports this notion. There also is evidence that estrogen is protective from heart disease. Although women's risk factors for heart disease climb after menopause, women's rate of death from heart attack and stroke do not equal that of men until women reach their 80s and 90s.

Why does this happen?[86] About 25% of estrogen's benefit is believed to be due to its effects on the metabolism of cholesterol. Estrogen helps metabolize fats that are eaten with meals and encourages some of the potentially more harmful remnants to be eliminated from the body more rapidly.[87] Also, more information came from the large Postmenopausal Estrogen/Progestin Interventions (PEPI) trial, a study that was done in women of average risk for heart disease who did not have heart disease at the time they were enrolled in the study. The PEPI study found that estrogen also increases high-density lipoprotein (HDL) cholesterol (good cholesterol) by about 10% and lowers bad, or low-density lipoprotein (LDL) cholesterol by about 10%.[88] Estrogen also increases the flow of blood through the heart's blood vessels and helps to keep them more elastic, even if there is atherosclerosis. This ability of estrogen may contribute up to 70% of its beneficial effects.[89] Soy also makes blood vessels more elastic. Unfortunately, estrogen does not lower triglycerides and may actually increase them if estrogen is taken by mouth as opposed to a patch.

Many of the benefits to the heart that are seen with estrogen also are seen in women who take combined estrogen/progesterone HRT. But research in animals has shown that progestins reduce the ability of estrogen to reduce plaque buildup in the blood vessels.[90] The higher the dosage of progesterone, the more this protection is reduced.

Because HRT seemed to protect the heart, it was thought that it might reduce the risk of heart attack and death in women who already had heart disease. That was the purpose of the Heart and Estrogen/Progestin Replacement Study (HERS). A total of 2,763 postmenopausal women (mean age 67 years) with established heart disease were randomly given either conjugated equine estrogen (i.e., Premarin) (CEE) with medroxyprogesterone acetate or a placebo. Over the next 4.1 years, the HRT group had an 11% decrease in LDL cholesterol and a 10% increase in HDL cholesterol compared with the placebo group. However, even though these cholesterol changes were extremely positive, the number of heart attacks was the same in both groups.[91] But after 4 years, things changed. Women taking HRT were less likely to have a heart attack than those women not getting it.

The Estrogen Replacement and Atherosclerosis (ERA) study was designed to compare CEE with CEE/medroxyprogesterone acetate and with a placebo. About 300 women who had narrowing of their arteries were enrolled to see if HRT had any effect on their disease.[92] Once again, if the disease was already present, HRT offered no improvement over taking a placebo.

At the present time, there is another study under way, which is not yet completed. It is called the HRT trial of the Women's Health Initiative from the National Heart, Lung, and Blood Institute.[93] After 2 years, the HRT group had a tendency to have more heart attacks than the placebo group, although the total number of women that had a heart attack was less than 1% and this number was not statistically significant. Because the information did not conclusively prove that HRT was harmful, it is still continuing and the results will be available in the next few years.

The bottom line on HRT and heart disease is if you are healthy and do not have heart disease, estrogen is probably protective and progesterone might reduce estrogen's benefits somewhat. If you already have heart disease or a history of blood clots, HRT may not be for you, especially medroxyprogesterone. Some authorities believe that estrogen is still okay, particularly if it is given as an injection, or as a gel, because giving it by these methods does not stimulate the liver to increase blood-clotting factors. You would still need to take another type of progesterone unless you have had a hysterectomy (uterus removed). Be sure what symptoms you are treating, understand your alternatives, and work with your doctor to individualize your treatment.

For instance, if your primary reason for taking estrogen is to prevent heart disease and your blood cholesterol levels are too high, discuss with your doctor the possibility of taking one of a number of cholesterol-lowering drugs called statins. They come under a variety of brand names such as Mevacor (lovastatin), Pravachol (pravastatin), Zocor (simvastatin), Lescol (fluvastatin), Lipitor (atorvastatin), and Baycol (cerivastatin). They can lower cholesterol levels by as much as 60% and the risk of fatal heart attacks by as much as 30% to 40%.[94] Recent studies raise the possibility of added benefits. They may also lower the risk of osteoporosis and reduce the chances of developing both Alzheimer's disease and other forms of dementia.[95] Add soy to your diet to control your hot flashes and you have created a terrific alternative plan.

HRT and Weight Gain

Although many women are certain they gained weight because they took estrogen, not one study supports this notion. What does happen as a result of aging is a slowing down of your metabolism. That means to maintain weight a woman should eat 3% to 5% less each decade of life whether or not she takes estrogen. If your only reason for saying no to estrogen is fear of gaining weight, stop worrying and take the estrogen.

HOW HRT IS PRESCRIBED

A woman who decides to take HRT still has two decisions to make. The first is which HRT regimen to use; the second is which specific estrogen and/or progesterone formulation to take. The first part of this decision can be decided easily by answering one question: Do you still want to have a period or not? Today there are three options for combining estrogen and progesterone: (1) sequential, which causes monthly bleeding; (2) continuous combined; and (3) intermittent. The last two options are intended to eliminate bleeding altogether. They are distinguished by the type of estrogen and progesterone used as well as by the dosing pattern of the progesterone choice.

The sequential regimen has been used for the longest period of time and is intended to mimic what happens during a menstrual cycle. Estrogen is given every day and progesterone is added for the last 10 to 14 days of each month of treatment. This will cause predictable bleeding resembling a normal period, although it may be lighter. This method, like the ones below, is similar to a birth control pill and prevents pregnancy as well as providing HRT. The bleeding does not mean you are ovulating again.

FIGURE 2-2. HRT OPTIONS

| ESTROGEN = Days of estrogen | PROGESTERONE = Days of progesterone |

Sequential	PROGESTERONE * PROGEST ESTROGEN* ESTROGEN*ESTROGEN*ESTROGEN*E
Continuous- Combined	PROGESTERONE * PROGESTERONE * PROGESTERON ESTROGEN* ESTROGEN*ESTROGEN*ESTROGEN*E
Daily Estrogen/ Intermittent Progestin (3 days on, 3 days off)	PROG PROG PROG PROG ESTROGEN* ESTROGEN*ESTROGEN*ESTROGEN*E

Days of the Month

The continuous-combined regimen uses a daily regimen of both estrogen and progesterone throughout the month. This is a good method to try, if the goal is to eliminate bleeding altogether. The uterine lining is kept thin, so that after a few months to 1 year of treatment, bleeding is greatly reduced or eliminated. If you are a few years into perimenopause rather than just starting it, it is more likely that you will stop bleeding.

The intermittent regimen is the newest. It really is a variation of the continuous-combined regimen, but with a lower total amount of progesterone. As its name implies, the intermittent regimen alternates 3 days of estrogen alone with 3 days of estrogen and progesterone. The theory is that during the estrogen-only days, the uterine lining becomes more sensitized to progesterone. Adding progesterone for only a short time at a low dose can cause the uterine lining to become thin.[96] Time will tell if this method is comparable or superior to the continuous-combined regimen or if patients will like it better.

HRT Formulations in the United States

After deciding which HRT regimen to take, there is still one more decision. Which HRT formulation do you use? There are five combination HRT products available for oral administration in a single pill.

TABLE 2-4. ORAL HRT COMBINATION PRODUCTS

Trade Name	Regimen	Estrogen Dose	Progestin Dose
Activella	Continuous-combined	1 mg 17β-estradiol (17βE$_2$)	0.5 mg norethindrone acetate (NETA)
femhrt	Continuous-combined	5 μg ethinyl estradiol (EE)	1.0 mg NETA
ORTHO-PREFEST	Intermittent	1 mg 17β-estradiol (17βE$_2$)	90 μg norgestimate (NGM) 3 days off, 3 days on
PREMPRO	Continuous-combined	0.625 mg conjugated equine estrogens (CEEs)	2.5 or 5 mg medroxyprogesterone acetate (MPA)
PREMPHASE	Sequential	0.625 mg CEE daily	5 mg MPA days 15–28

NOTE: μg = microgram; mg = milligram.
SOURCE: Package inserts.

In addition to these pharmaceutical preparations, there are also a number of "natural" estrogen preparations. It is important to understand that these "natural" substances are also made in pharmaceutical plants rather than botanical plants. They are natural in that they are compounded to include ratios of the body's three principal estrogens (estrone or E1, estradiol or E2, and estriol or E3) in ratios that are typically found in women. The most common brand is Tri-Estrogen or Tri-Est for short, because it contains E1, E2, and E3. A similar product called Bi-Est contains E2 and E3. These estrogens are usually available by prescription only in compounding drugstores and not the traditional chain drugstores.[97] Tri-Est was developed in the early 1980s by Jonathan Wright, M.D., and contains 80% estriol, 10% estradiol, and 10% estrone. Bi-Est contains 80% E3 and 20% E2. They are available as capsules, topical creams and gels, sublingual drops, vaginal creams, suppositories, and lozenges. They do not come as a patch.

The gel can be applied once or twice daily by rubbing a quarter of a teaspoon onto the face, neck, or brow or onto the inner side of the arms and forearms. Absorption from the abdomen and inner thigh might be less. Capsules are absorbed best with meals, preferably ones that contain fat in them, and come in strengths ranging from 0.625 to 2.5 mg. Three or four sublingual drops (not dropperfuls) containing 0.625 mg of estrogen per drop (0.0625 mg of estrone, 0.0625 mg of estradiol, and 0.5 mg of estriol) are applied under the tongue twice daily and allowed to absorb rather than be swallowed. Vaginal creams or gels that do not contain alcohol (which can be irritating) typically contain estriol only, 1 to 2 mg per gram of cream.

Estriol is the most abundant estrogen produced by the placenta. It has become the natural estrogen of choice among the alternative women's health advocates because they believe it is safe. Some alternative-drug catalogs specifically state that estriol prevents cancer of the breast and uterine lining. There is some basis for these claims, but unfortunately, there are no studies in which estriol was given to women as protection to support such claims.

There are studies showing that pretreatment with estriol limits the rate of breast tumors in rats fed carcinogens.[98] Estriol also has been found to shrink breast tumors in rats and humans.[99] However, before we become too excited about this, we have to remember that diethylstilbestrol (DES), estrone, and estradiol have all been used at one time to treat breast cancer, and each of them has been able to cause a short-term remission.

There are also some observational studies that suggest estriol is protective against cancer. Women who have their first baby early in life excrete more estriol than women who have never had a baby. Having your first baby early seems to be protective against breast cancer. Asian women, who have a lower rate of breast cancer than their American counterparts, excrete more estriol than American women. As Asian women adopt a more American way of life, their estriol excretion decreases and their breast cancer rates rise.[100] Of course, this change in breast cancer rates may also reflect the fact that Asians who adopt more Western diets are eating less soy in their diets.

The evidence for estriol being protective against breast cancer in premenopausal women seems good. But after menopause the story changes. High estriol levels in postmenopausal women suggests that the body is making high levels of estrogen, which is associated with an increased risk of breast cancer.[101] Estriol is a weaker estrogen than estradiol, and some practitioners feel it protects the uterine lining from developing cancer. This is not true. Estriol is just as likely to cause the uterine lining to go through precancerous changes as estradiol, if it is given at comparable dosages.[102] The studies that suggested it protected the uterine lining were performed using less than adequate dosages of estriol. Estriol has limitations: It does not prevent bone loss[103] and it does not bind to LDL, or bad cholesterol. Therefore it has no antioxidant activity. However, it does help reduce hot flashes.

Estrone tablets (Ogen, a purified crystalline form of estrone sulfate) come in dosages of 0.625-, 1.25-, and 2.5-mg tablets, as well as in a vaginal cream, all by prescription (see Table 2-5). The 0.625-mg dosage is able to lower total cholesterol whether or not it is taken together with medroxyprogesterone acetate.[104] The role of estrone alone, for other reasons, is less well studied.

To summarize: "Natural" estrogens are not really natural. They are made in pharmaceutical plants rather than botanical plants. But they are compounded to include ratios of the body's three principal estrogens (estrone or E1, estradiol or E2, and estriol or E3) in ratios that are typically found in women. They may also be prescribed individually. The benefits of "natural" estrogens appear largely due to estradiol, although estrone seems to be able to lower cholesterol. If you use estriol alone, you'll likely need to combine it with either another estrogen or alternative agents to protect your heart and bones. The risks of natural estrogens have not been nearly as well studied as those of conju-

gated equine estrogens, but are likely to be the same if comparable dosages are given.

Alternative Routes for Taking Estrogen

INTRAVAGINAL CREAMS

Many women think that vaginal estrogen stays only in the
vagina. In fact, vaginal estrogens are well absorbed into the
bloodstream. Women who are having a particular problem with
upset stomach taking estrogen find vaginal creams a big
improvement. In addition to Tri-Est, which was mentioned
above, several other intravaginal estrogens are also available (see
Table 2-5). Ogen, Estrace, Premarin, and Ortho Dienestrol vaginal creams, and Estring vaginal ring can all be substituted for
oral estrogen. Because they are absorbed through the vagina and
not through the intestinal tract, they are not metabolized by the
liver. So the actual amount available to your body is even greater
than if you took the same dosage orally. However, because each
of these preparations has different estrogen doses that are not
equivalent, it is necessary to measure the amount of estradiol in
your blood to be certain that the amount you are given is in the
therapeutic range. In addition to the vaginal creams and the
estrogen ring, there is also a vaginal gel tablet (Vagifem).

SKIN CREAMS AND GELS

Estrogen can also be applied through the skin as a cream or gel.
In addition to the Tri-Est listed above, compounding pharmacies
often produce their own versions. Be aware: Potency and reliability may vary greatly from one batch to another and from one
pharmacist to another.

Some of these gels are used widely in Europe and in tests performed they have been found to be as effective as oral estrogen in
relieving hot flashes.[105] One commonly used European prepara-

TABLE 2-5. INTRAVAGINAL ESTROGEN PREPARATIONS

Brand	Estrogen	Content
Ogen	Estropipate (purified estrone)	1.5 mg/g
Premarin	Conjugated equine estrogens	0.625 mg/g
Estrace	Estradiol	0.1 mg/g
Ortho Dienestrol	Dienestrol	0.01 mg/g
Vagifem vaginal gel tablet	Estradiol hemihydrate	25.8 µg = 25 µg of estradiol
Estring vaginal ring	Estradiol	2 mg per ring releases 7.5 µg/24 hours for 90 days

SOURCE: Modified from *Menopause Guidebook*. North American Menopause Society, 2001. Dosages from package inserts.

tion contains 1.5 mg of estradiol applied in 2.5 grams of gel each day. It is applied to both arms over an area of about 800 square centimeters (cm²), which is roughly 10 square inches. This dosage helps reduce hot flashes and is as effective against osteoporosis as 0.625 mg of Premarin daily.[106] With the gel preparations, it is possible to get too much as well as too little estrogen. So if you use them be sure to have your estrogen level checked, either in blood or saliva, to be certain you are absorbing a therapeutic amount. If your level is either too high or too low, have your estrogen level repeated again in a month or so to be sure you are in an acceptable range. See your doctor for a blood test, or mail in a saliva sample to one of the salivary test centers easily found on the internet (*www.aeron.com.* or *www.salivatest.com*).

PROGESTERONE AND PROGESTINS

Progesterone is the hormone of ovulation. The ovary produces it each month after the egg is released to prepare the uterine lining for conception and to help sustain a pregnancy. Progesterone also keeps the menstrual cycle regular and normal and balances estrogen's potential negative effects on the body. Progesterone also plays a role in protecting the breast and uterus from developing cancer. It increases HDL, or good cholesterol, improves the breakdown of fat into energy, and cuts the body's craving for carbohydrates and sweets. In fact, progesterone deficiency is commonly a cause of premenstrual syndrome (PMS) symptoms and painful, lumpy breasts.[107]

Sometimes progesterone, which is a naturally occurring hormone, is confused with the synthetic class of hormones called progestins or progestogens. They are quite different. Progestins are patented, chemically modified molecules that in the body act similar to progesterone. They are also responsible for many of the side effects attributed to progesterone. There are two principal types of progestins. Provera (medroxyprogesterone acetate) and similar generic products are chemical alterations of the progesterone molecule and are called 17-hydroxyprogesterones. The other type of progestin is actually a chemical alteration of testosterone called 19-nortestosterones.

Types of Progesterones

NATURAL

- Suppositories
- Micronized powder
- Progestasert IUD
- Prometrium
- Crinone 4% and 8%
- Pro-Gest (nonprescription)

SYNTHETIC

17-Hydroxyprogesterones (progestins that contain 17 or 21 carbon atoms)
- Medroxyprogesterone acetate
- Megastrol acetate

- Cyproterone acetate
- Dydrogesterone
- Medrogestone

19-Nortestosterone (progestins that contain 19 carbon atoms)
- Norethindrone acetate (NETA)
- Norethindrone
- Ethynodiol diacetate
- Lynestrenol
- Norgestrel, levo norgestrel (LNg)
- Desogestrel
- Norgestimate (NGM)

SELECTIVE ESTROGEN RECEPTOR MODULATORS

In several places throughout this book we have discussed estrogen receptors—tiny docking stations on the surface of or within the body of cells that estrogen must attach to for it to cause a biologic effect. As I have explained, there are two types of estrogen receptors—alpha and beta. The breasts and uterus have mainly alpha receptors. Bones and the cardiovascular system have mainly beta receptors. Estradiol attaches to both alpha and beta receptors. SERMs are a group of medicines similar to estrogen, with one exception: They were designed to selectively avoid stimulating the alpha estrogen receptors on the breast and uterus. That is why they have been given the nickname "smart estrogens." There are four SERMs approved by the FDA for different indications. Here are their names and what they are approved for:

Tamoxifen (Nolvadex)

- Early breast cancer treatment along with other forms of therapy
- Healthy women at high risk for breast cancer

- First-line treatment for metastatic breast cancer that is estrogen receptor positive

Raloxifene (Evista)

- Osteoporosis

Toremifene (Fareston)

- First-line treatment for metastatic breast cancer that is estrogen receptor positive

Clomiphene citrate (Clomid, Serophene)

- Approved for the treatment of faulty ovulation

A more complete list of SERMs and the parent compounds they are derived from is given below:

Triphenylethylenes

- Clomiphene
- Tamoxifen
- Toremifene
- Droloxifene
- Idoxifene

Benzothiophenes

- Raloxifene
- LY353381

Naphthalenes

- CP336,156

Chromans

- Levormeloxifene

Phytoestrogens

- Genistein
- Daidzein

Conjugated Estrogens

- Delta 8,9-dehydroestrone sulfate

Each SERM has a different activity depending on how it is structured. Differences in structure cause differences in how a SERM works in the body. For instance, one SERM may stimulate the growth of bone and, at the same time, block the effect of estrogen on the breast. When a SERM changes the shape of the receptor so estrogen cannot affect the cell, it is called an antiestrogen or estrogen antagonist for that particular tissue. If the SERM fits into the estrogen receptor and causes the effects that estrogen would, it is called an estrogen agonist for that tissue. Ideally, a SERM would stop hot flashes, protect against osteoporosis, heart disease, and Alzheimer's disease, and not increase the risk of breast or uterine cancer. When we look at the two most widely used SERMs, tamoxifen and raloxifene, we can see that they do not meet these goals perfectly. We can also see that isoflavones found in soy (genistein and daidzein) are more selective for beta receptors and come pretty close to being an ideal SERM.

TABLE 2-6. BIOLOGICAL ACTIVITY OF ESTROGEN, SERMS, AND ISOFLAVONES

	Brain	Uterus	Vagina	Breast	Bone	Heart
Estradiol	++	++	++	++	++	++
Pure antiestrogen	--	--	--	--	--	--
Ideal SERM	++	--	++	--	++	++
Tamoxifen	--	+	--	--	+	+
Raloxifene	--	--	--	--	+	+
Isoflavones	+	--	+/-	+/-	+	+

Clinical Uses of SERMs

TAMOXIFEN

As shown above, tamoxifen is only used in women with early breast cancer or in those at high risk for getting it. It acts as an antiestrogen in breast tissue, but it can act like estrogen on the uterine lining and cause polyps and even cancers.[108] The antiestrogen effects of tamoxifen caused it to be approved in the United States in 1977 for the treatment of advanced breast cancer in postmenopausal women.[109] Tamoxifen was approved in 1985 to be used together with chemotherapy in postmenopausal women who had breast cancer that had spread to the lymph nodes. In 1989, tamoxifen was approved for use in premenopausal women with advanced breast cancer that could be proven to have estrogen receptors on it. In 1990, tamoxifen was approved to treat advanced breast cancer whether or not the lymph nodes were involved if there were estrogen receptors on the cancer cells. Since 1998, tamoxifen has been approved to prevent breast cancer in women at high risk for the disease.

Tamoxifen may have some other benefits. It slows down the rate of bone loss and offers some protection against osteoporosis.[110] Tamoxifen also seems to improve cholesterol levels in women who take it. Women who use tamoxifen should have an ultrasound of their uterine lining done each year to be certain that the medication is not causing polyps or uterine cancer. There is also an increased risk of blood clots both in the legs (deep vein thrombosis) and to the lung (pulmonary embolism), hot flashes, and developing cataracts (clouding of the lens of the eye) while taking this medication. If you are not at high risk of developing breast cancer, do not take tamoxifen for breast-cancer prevention. Also do not take it for more than 5 years. Women who do may actually increase their risk of breast cancer.

RALOXIFENE

Like tamoxifen, raloxifene was originally developed as a treatment for advanced breast cancer. It does help prevent breast cancer, but more studies must be done before we know for certain that it is an effective medication for this purpose. The Study of Tamoxifen and Raloxifene (STAR) trial was begun by the National Cancer Institute in 1999 and will last for 5 to 10 years. It will be the largest breast-cancer-prevention study ever conducted and involve over 300 different clinics from all over the United States, Canada, and Puerto Rico.

Raloxifene has been approved for the treatment of osteoporosis in postmenopausal women since December 1997. The dosage is usually 60 mg per day. Although it does prevent bone loss, it does not do so as well as conjugated equine estrogen.[111] Raloxifene lowers total cholesterol, LDL cholesterol (bad cholesterol), and triglycerides, but it does not increase the amount of HDL cholesterol (good cholesterol). Raloxifene causes leg cramps and increases hot flashes in some women.[112] If you are taking raloxifene and suffer from hot flashes while taking it, try adding soy to your diet or soy isoflavone tablets.

* * *

To summarize: Evaluating the risks and benefits of HRT is not easy, particularly in light of the July 2002 Women's Health Initiative study and the National Cancer Institute study published the same month. The risks of estrogen alone are still being evaluated in a continuing WHI study. However, the risks of estrogen plus progesterone, in particular medroxyprogesterone, appear worrisome in reference to blood clots and breast cancer. But even in that study the risk of hip fracture and colon cancer declined. Even "smart" estrogens can create problems and are not for everyone. Once again and most important, know why you would take estrogen, weigh the risks and benefits, and understand what other alternatives you have. While you are sorting all of this out with your doctor, pick up some soy and start getting some of its benefits.

chapter 3

SOY BASICS

A BRIEF HISTORY OF NUTRITION

Hippocrates wrote extensively on the relationship between nutrition and health around 400 B.C. Dioscorides, a Greek physician who lived before Hippocrates, described some 600 plants possessing medicinal properties, including many that are still being used today. The Greek philosophers Pythagoras and Plato advocated a vegetarian diet to promote health, and the Greek physician Galen developed specific food treatments around A.D. 130.[1]

In the early twentieth century scientists discovered that food contained fat, water, carbohydrates, proteins, minerals, and a sixth class of food elements called vitamins. In 1912 Casimir Funk coined the term "vital amine" to describe those organic compounds that must be included in the human diet in order to maintain normal health. The word vitamin is a later evolution of this phrase.[2]

The discovery of vitamins helped explain many lessons that were learned from observation. For example, James Lind, a ship's doctor with the British Royal Navy in 1747, found that fruits and vegetables rich in vitamin C cured sailors who contracted scurvy, a disease that causes bleeding gums, muscle weakness, and eventually death. In the early 1900s, beriberi, a disease that attacks the nerves, heart, and digestive system, was cured by thiamin. Similarly, in 1938, pellagra, a disease characterized by dermatitis, diarrhea, dementia, and death, was found to be cured by niacin. It was not until 1982 that the National Academy of Sciences, on behalf of the National Cancer Institute, issued a report recommending that we eat more fruits and vegetables. In that report, the National Academy highlighted the importance of phytochemicals. The prefix "phyto" means plant. Phytochemicals are components of foods that are not nutrients but do affect health.

This book is about the many positive health benefits of soy. As you read on you will learn how soy and the phytochemicals it contains can help to reduce hot flashes, lower your risk of heart disease and osteoporosis, and possibly even lower the risk of certain cancers. I cannot emphasize enough how important it is to realize that many of the common diseases found in prosperous nations today could potentially be avoided by significantly modifying diet.[3] By that I mean eating less in general to reduce the health risks that come with being overweight, and eating less animal fats and refined sugars while increasing the consumption of fruits, vegetables, and plant foods, particularly foods like soy.

A SHORT HISTORY OF SOY

The history of the soybean is an ancient one, beginning over five thousand years ago in eastern Asia where it grew wild on vines. Chinese farmers cultivated these wild vines and called them *tatou,* which means "greater bean."[4] The Japanese call soy sauce *shoyu.* Some time around 1600 B.C. the Chinese literature referred to soybeans as *sou.* Our term soy could have come from either of these terms. The soybean was so important to the ancient Chinese that the Chinese emperor Sheng-Nung mentioned soybeans in his *Ben Tsao Gang Mu* in 2838 B.C., and listed it as one of five sacred crops. Over time, the domesticated soybean spread throughout Asia to Korea, Japan, and Southeast Asia. It took much longer to travel to Europe, where it finally arrived around the eighteenth century.

How soy got to the West is still uncertain. Some theorize that European sailors used bags of soybeans as ballast on return trips from China. Others speculate that European traders and missionaries brought it back with them from Asia. It seems to have come to the United States with the Chinese immigrants who settled here.

Doctors Messina and Setchell point out the important role Dr. John Harvey Kellogg of corn flakes fame played in popularizing soy.[5] As an ardent supporter of vegetarianism, he used his Battle Creek sanatorium to invent granola as a substitute for bacon and eggs. Kellogg invented breakfast cereals, as we know them, and gave Americans their first soymilk and meat substitutes made from soy. Dr. Kellogg was influenced by Ellen White, founder of the Seventh-Day Adventist Church, whose members are usually vegetarian. She advocated the use of meat substitutes "so that meat will not be desired." To this day many studies on soy are conducted at medical schools affiliated with the Seventh-Day Adventist Church. Through their work and the efforts of many others around the world, the humble soybean has gone from zero to hero as thousands of scientific studies conducted on soy over the past two decades have helped explain its many health benefits.

GENES AND BEANS

Because it is expected that the world's population will double to more than 10 billion people during our children's lifetime, there is a growing need to provide food and fiber to feed and clothe these many people.[6] It has become possible to modify plants by adding genetic material to change them slightly, with the intention of improving the world's food supply. In North America in 2001, more than 57 million acres of a variety of plants had been treated this way, including soybeans, potatoes, corn, tomatoes, and others, up from 4 million acres in 1996.[7] Plants changed in this way are called GMO or genetically modified organism. In the case of soy, the goal is to insert a small piece of genetic material into the bean so that a particular weed killer will not affect it. This allows the farmer to spray the weeds with small amounts of the weed killer and know the soy plant will be immune. It is believed that the only thing changed in the plant is the ability to tolerate the weed killer. Soybeans treated this way will yield about 5% more soy on the same amount of land. At the same time less weed killer needs to be used.

Many issues have been raised about GMO plants in our food system and in our society. Some strongly favor the process and feel it is both safe and will help feed the world. Others fear that GMO plants may alter naturally growing plants or cause other problems. I am not aware of any reports of GMO soy having a bad effect on people. However, by error, a GMO brand of corn intended for animal food was mistakenly made into taco shells and caused food allergy in a number of people. More studies have to be done before we can know the impact of GMO foods. Foods that have not been altered in any way are called GMO free.

A BOTANICAL DESCRIPTION

Scientists call the soybean *Glycine max* and classify it as a member of the legume family. Domesticated soy plants grow to about two feet tall. They have a woody stem with broad leaves, with flowers and seed pods. The pods look like snap beans, except that as the soybean develops, the leaves, stems, and growing pods are covered with soft brownish-green hairs. Each seed pod is typically 1½ to 2 inches long and contains two to three beans. Asian soybeans are typically a little larger than those grown in the United States and Canada. When they are fresh, soybeans look a lot like green peas. The immature pods are harvested early in July and sold while they are still green.[8] The remainder of the crop is harvested in the fall after the plants have lost their leaves and the mature beans have dried on the vine. By then they usually have taken on a yellow-beige color, although some are green, purple, brown, black, or even spotted.

Soybeans are not only good for people, they are actually good for the soil as well. Most crops must be rotated; planted with different crops every few years, so that the soil will remain fertile. Soy actually enriches the soil it is grown in. That is because soy, like other legumes, is an important part of the nitrogen cycle. Nitrogen makes up about 78% of the earth's atmosphere and all living things require it. But most organisms cannot use nitrogen gas. Soy is able to remove nitrogen from the atmosphere and turn it into amino acids, the building blocks of proteins. Soy also contains nitrogen-fixing bacteria that can remove nitrogen from the atmosphere and turn it into nitrogen-containing organic substances that it puts back into the soil. This enriches the land and allows it to be used over and over again without rotation. Here is how it works. The soybean plant secretes a plant hormone called genistein into the soil (more about genistein later). The genistein chemically attracts the bacteria *Bradyrhizobium* sp, which stimulate the soy plant to make special sugars that cause the soy plant to make nodules on its roots that house these bacteria. These root nodules are the sites where atmospheric nitrogen is converted into nitrogen that is put back into the soil.[9] Some call soy "green manure." This rich source of nitrogen is also important for people, which we will discuss later.

A POWERFUL SOURCE OF PROTEIN

Soy has many health benefits, and it is a terrific source of nutrition. Nearly two hundred years ago, when scientists discovered the significance of protein to our diet, they gave it a name based on the Greek word *proteios,* which means "of prime importance." The enzymes that help digest food and assemble or divide molecules to make new cells and chemical substances to control metabolism are made of protein. Many important hormones, such as insulin, which helps us to utilize the sugar we eat, and gonadotropins that regulate reproduction, also are made of proteins. Proteins make up our hair, our nails, and the outer layers of our skin, the clear fluid in blood called plasma, the rubbery inner structure of our bones, and part of our muscles. Proteins are such a major building block of our bodies that if we got rid of all the water in our body, half of the remaining weight would be pure protein.

Understanding Proteins

Proteins are long molecules that contain carbon, hydrogen, and oxygen atoms plus a nitrogen (amino) group. Proteins are our only source of nitrogen, which is essential for synthesizing specialized proteins in our bodies. Think of proteins as long chains made up of small links called amino acids. These amino acids are the basic building blocks of all proteins. There are twenty-two different amino acids. Thirteen are nonessential—if we do not eat them in our food, we can manufacture them from carbohydrates, fats, and other amino acids. But nine are essential, meaning we cannot synthesize them in our bodies, and we must get them from food.

ESSENTIAL AMINO ACIDS

- Phenylalanine
- Lysine
- Isoleucine
- Methionine
- Threonine
- Leucine
- Tryptophan
- Valine
- Histidine

NONESSENTIAL AMINO ACIDS

- Glycine
- Glutamic acid
- Proline
- Alanine
- Serine
- Hydroxyproline
- Cystine
- Citrulline
- Tyrosine
- Arginine
- Aspartic acid
- Norleucine
- Hydroxyglutamic acid

As you might expect, foods vary in the amount and variety of amino acids that they contain. Most proteins of animal origin contain proteins that are similar in combination to human protein, which is why meat, fish, poultry, eggs, and dairy products are called high-quality proteins. Most plant proteins—grains, fruit, vegetables, legumes (beans), nuts, and seeds—do not contain the entire list of essential amino acids, so their nutritional quality is less valuable to us. The major exception is soy. Soybeans contain all nine essential amino acids, which makes them an excellent source of proteins for vegetarians and especially for vegans—vegetarians who avoid all animal products including milk and eggs. Soy protein has another important advantage—it is easily broken down by our digestive enzymes.

Soybeans also contain a high percentage of their volume as protein. Most beans contain 20% protein by volume, but soybeans contain 40%. Soy is an excellent source of protein compared to beef and wheat. Consider a farmer who uses an acre of land to produce protein: If he raised a cow on one acre of land, it would contain enough protein for one person for 77 days. If he used that same acre of land and grew wheat, there would be enough protein to sustain one person for 877 days. However, if he decided to grow soy on the same one acre of land, there would be enough protein produced to sustain one person for 2,224 days.

How Much Protein Do We Really Need?

Adults need only about 0.8 gram of protein per day for every kilogram (kg), or 2.2 pounds, of their body weight, which is slightly more than 0.4 gram for every pound.[10] Infants (up to 2 grams/kg per day), adolescents (1.2 grams/kg per day), and pregnant women (10-plus grams/kg per day and 12–15 grams/kg per day if nursing), and people with injuries, burns, or bone fractures need slightly more.

How much does the average person need? A 138-pound

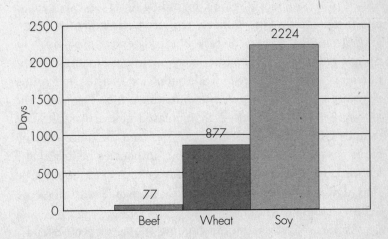

Protein Yield/Acre/Person

FIGURE 3-1.   Average Amount of Protein Given for One Person per Acre

woman needs about 50 grams of protein a day and a 175-pound man, about 64 grams. This would be about two to three 3-ounce servings of lean meat, fish, or chicken (21 grams of protein each). According to Carol Ann Rinzler, a noted authority on nutrition, a vegetarian equivalent would be 2 eggs (12 to 16 grams), 2 slices of prepacked fat-free cheese (10 grams), 4 slices of bread (3 grams each), and 1 cup of yogurt (10 grams). A vegan could accomplish the same protein intake by eating a cup of tofu (20 grams) and one-half cup of dry roasted soybeans (34 grams), or 2 to 3 ounces of soy protein concentrate (22.6 grams each). As you can see, protein deficiency in the United States is unlikely. In this country, most people are eating far more protein than they need.

Does eating more protein than we need cause a problem? Over time, the answer is yes. The extra protein we eat must either be burned for calories or turned into fat. There is an additional problem when extra protein calories come from animal protein—they bring into our bodies extra doses of saturated fats and cholesterol. Both of these substances have been linked to a variety of diseases, including heart disease, cancer, and osteoporosis. Our kidneys, too, are overworked by excess animal protein. Kidney disease is a progressive problem. The normal kidney works as a filter, keeping in our bloodstream the nutrients that we need while allowing waste and other unwanted material to pass out into the urine. The more the kidney has to filter (called an increased glomerular filtration rate, or GFR), the harder it has to work and the more vulnerable it is to becoming diseased. Some authorities believe that a low-protein diet, especially one that includes soy, could even slow down the rate of kidney disease in people with diabetes. Table 3-1 shows why.

As you see, soy is an outstanding source of protein and a ready source of food to feed the hungry people of the world.

TABLE 3-1. EFFECT OF PROTEIN TYPE ON GLOMERULAR FILTRATION RATE

Protein	Percent Increase in GFR
Beef	50
Chicken	35
Fish	20
Soy	None

OTHER NUTRITIONAL BENEFITS OF SOY

Although soy is clearly a fabulous source of protein, from a nutritional point of view it is also much more (see Figure 3-2). As I've mentioned before, soy contains no cholesterol, and it is a rich source of vitamins and minerals. There are literally hundreds of soy foods to choose from. Some of the more common ones are listed in Figure 3-2. I've taken selections from what is available on the USDA Nutrient Database for Standard Reference (*www.nal.usda.gov/fnic/cgi-bin/nut_search.p1*). If you want either more information on the soy foods listed below or you want to know the specific nutritional details of other soy foods, just go to the Web site, type in the food by name, or type in a specific NDB number if you have it.

"Vitamin S" and Minerals Too

Soybeans are such a rich source of important vitamins and minerals that I sometimes think of soy as "vitamin S." Soy is a particularly good source of the B complex vitamins, which include folic acid and vitamin B_6 along with thiamin (B_1), riboflavin (B_2), niacin (B_3), and pantothenic acid (B_5).

Everyone knows that too much cholesterol can contribute to heart disease. But another important substance that may be just

FIGURE 3-2. NUTRITIONAL VALUE OF SOY FOODS

Soy Food	Protein (g)	Fat (g)	Carbo-hydrate (g)	Fiber (g)	Calcium (mg)	Sodium (mg)	Iron (mg)	Zinc (mg)	Thiamin (mg)	Riboflavin (mg)	Niacin (mg)	Vitamin B_6 (mg)	Folate (mcg)
Soybeans boiled, 1 cup	22.23	11.52	19.89	7.56	261	450	4.5	1.638	0.468	0.279	2.25	0.108	199.8
Soybeans, dry roasted, 1 cup	68	37.2	56.2	9.2	464		6.8	8.2	0.8	1.4	1.8	0.38	351.8
Soy flour, low-fat, roasted, 1 cup	40.95	5.896	33.422	8.976	165.44	15.84	5.271	1.038	0.334	0.251	1.901	0.459	360.8
Soy flour, defatted, 1 cup	51.46	1.22	33.93	17.5	241	20	9.24	2.46	0.698	0.253	2.612	0.574	305.4
Soy Protein concentrate from alcohol extraction, 1 oz	16.48	0.13	8.8	1.6	103		3	0.09	0.09	0.04	0.203	0.038	96.39
Soy protein isolate, 1 oz	22.9	0.96	2.087	1.588	50.463	284.918	4.1	1.14	0.05	0.028	0.408	0.028	49.924
Soymilk, 1 cup	6.7	4.7	4.4	3.2	9.8	29.4	1.42	0.56	0.4	0.17	0.36	0.1	3.68
Miso, 1 cup	32.477	14.85	76.89	14.85	181.5	10029.25	7.535	9.13	0.267	0.688	2.365	.591	91.75

(continued)

FIGURE 3-2. NUTRITIONAL VALUE OF SOY FOODS (continued)

Soy Food	Protein (g)	Fat (g)	Carbo-hydrate (g)	Fiber (g)	Calcium (mg)	Sodium (mg)	Iron (mg)	Zinc (mg)	Thiamin (mg)	Riboflavin (mg)	Niacin (mg)	Vitamin B_6 (mg)	Folate (mcg)
Natto, 1 cup	31.01	19.25	25.113	9.45	379.75	12.25	15.05	5.303	0.28	0.333	0	0.228	14
Tofu, okara, 1 cup	3.928	2.111	15.299		97.6	10.98	1.586	0.683	0.024	0.024	0.122	0.14	32.208
Tempeh, 1 cup	30.776	17.928	15.597	N/A	184.26	14.94	4.487	1.892	0.129	0.594	4.382	0.357	39.674
Tofu, hard, w/nigari, ¼ block	15.47	12.188	5.356	0.732	420.9	2.44	3.355	2.025	0.051	0.094	0.78	0.048	26.84
Tofu, soft, w/CaSO4 & MgCl2 ¼ block	7.598	4.2	2.088	0.232	128.76	9.28	1.288	0.742	0.055	0.043	0.621	0.06	51.04

SOURCE: USDA Nutrient Database for Standard References, www.nal.usda.gov/fnic

as important in clogging arteries is homocysteine. B vitamins, in particular B_6 and folic acid, help the body to metabolize homocysteine to the amino acid methionine.[11] If people do not get enough of these essential B vitamins, homocysteine levels build up in the blood and act like Velcro. The homocysteine sticks to the blood vessel walls and cholesterol sticks to the homocysteine, which can lead to blood clots and even heart attacks. Soy can help provide enough B vitamins to keep homocysteine levels in the normal range.

Vitamin E was first discovered in soybeans. Having this natural antioxidant may be one of the ways that soy is helpful in fighting heart disease. Soy is also a rich source of calcium and magnesium. Later, in Chapter 10, we discuss incorporating soy into your diet. But now let me say a word about tofu. Tofu is curdled soymilk. It can be made in one of two ways: by adding nigari (which contains magnesium chloride), calcium sulfate, or both in varying quantities to precipitate the protein. Calcium and magnesium contents will vary accordingly and, depending on which are used, tofu can be a rich source of both of these important minerals.

Soy and Fiber

We hear a lot of talk about dietary fiber in relation to lowering cholesterol levels.[12] But did you realize that dietary fiber is a type of carbohydrate? Unlike simple carbohydrates that contain only one unit of sugar (monosaccharide) or two units of sugar (disaccharide), or complex carbohydrates that contain more than two units of sugar (polysaccharides), dietary fiber cannot be broken down by the human digestive system to be absorbed and used as a source of energy. The chemical bonds that hold its sugar units together are too strong. As dietary fiber passes through the small intestines of our digestive system, it either interferes with the absorption of cholesterol or with its metabolism. There are two types of fiber—soluble and insoluble. When soluble fiber passes into the colon, bacteria that live there can digest it by fermentation.[13] This is one way that soy helps to lower cholesterol. The average dietary recommendation is about 25 grams of fiber daily. The average American woman gets about half of that and the average American man gets slightly more at 17 grams.

Soy is a rich source of fiber. Half a cup of dry roasted soybeans has nearly 5 grams of fiber, which is nearly half of what the average American consumes. Use Figure 3-2 to find out the fiber content of different soy foods. Even one serving a day can help ensure your getting enough dietary fiber. Getting enough dietary fiber can lower cholesterol, which can help to battle heart disease. But there is another benefit. Dietary fiber forms gel in our intestinal tract when it mixes with water. This gel helps us feel full without eating as much and without absorbing as many calories because the fiber cannot be absorbed. It also helps to keep stools softer and bowel habits more regular, all extra benefits from eating soy.

Soy and Fats

Soy is also incredibly low in saturated fat—depending on the choice of soy food, 0% to 15% of fat contained in soybeans is saturated. About 62% of the fat in soybeans is unsaturated fatty acids and 23% monounsaturated. Neither of these unsaturated types of fatty acids increases cholesterol. Compare two tacos made from 4 ounces of extra lean beef versus a similar taco made from ½ cup of textured vegetable protein derived from soy. The one containing beef also has 18 grams of total fat of which 7.2 grams are saturated. The one made from soy has 0.1 gram of total fat and no saturated fat. You would also save about 200 calories.

Soy is also important because it is one of the few plant foods (along with olive and canola oils) that contain linolenic acid, which is an omega-3 fatty acid and the type of healthy fat that is primarily found in fish.[14] Our bodies are able to take the linolenic acid found in soy and process it into gamma-linolenic acid (GLA) that is an omega-3 fatty acid similar to the heart-healthy ones found in fish oil.[15] Many studies have shown that omega-3 fatty acids help to reduce the risk of heart disease. They also play an important role in the brain development of growing infants. In Chapter 6 (Soy and Heart Disease) we will talk more about fats.

OTHER SUBSTANCES FOUND IN SOY

Saponins

Saponins are glycosides—compounds made from sugars. They can be found in other plants besides soy, but they do not come from animal proteins. Saponins foam in water, which make them useful as emulsifying agents. Emulsifying agents keep water and fats mixed together in foods. They are also used in detergents and household products.

Saponins also play a role in biology. They have the ability to free hemoglobin from red blood cells, which helps to carry oxygen to the lungs. They have also been found to work as an anti-inflammatory agent with an action similar to cortisone. The saponins in soy may play a role in lowering cholesterol, either by blocking it from being absorbed or by causing more cholesterol to be eliminated from the intestinal tract. Saponins may also play a role in fighting cancer.[16] Not everyone agrees on how important the role of saponins is in our overall health.

Phytosterols

Phytosterols are so similar to cholesterol that they compete for absorption within the intestines. The end result is that less cholesterol gets absorbed.[17] In one large review of 80 studies on phytosterols, the authors concluded that the beneficial effects not only included lowering cholesterol but also in fighting tumors.[18] In one study published in the *New England Journal of Medicine*, the soy phytosterol sitostanol was used to make a margarine that was able to lower cholesterol levels more than 10% over the course of one year.[19] Phytosterols are believed to play a role in protecting against cancer, and are found in soy and in other plants.

Lecithin

Soy oil has high levels of lecithin (from the Greek, meaning "egg yolk"). Like saponins, lecithins are emulsifying agents and are used in food products. Without lecithin it would be difficult to keep the fat and water in ice cream together and the whole carton would be a sticky mess. It is used to smooth out chocolates and margarines and also has many nonfood applications, such as skin creams. Like other components of soy, lecithin may play a role in lowering cholesterol, but the amount we would have to eat is probably too great for it to be widely used. The average American intake of lecithin is about 3 grams per day, and the amount needed to lower cholesterol is estimated to be 2 to 10 times that amount.[20]

One important substance derived from lecithin is choline. In April 1998, choline was classified as an essential nutrient for humans.[21] It is the precursor of phosphatidylcholine and sphingomyelin, two substances that are necessary to protect nerve tissue. Choline is present in high amounts in eggs, liver, peanuts, many meats, cauliflower, and as you might have guessed, soybeans.

Choline is particularly important during pregnancy. Getting enough of it during that time appears to help babies have better memories and attention spans. Choline may also be important in preventing memory loss after menopause.[22]

UNDERSTANDING PHYTOESTROGENS, ISOFLAVONES, AND A LOT MORE

In order to understand some of the health benefits of soy, we have to discuss a little bit of plant biochemistry. Let's start with phytochemicals. The prefix "phyto" means plant, so phytochemicals are natural compounds that come from plants. Phytoestrogens is a name given to a broad group of plant compounds that have a chemical structure similar to estrogen, which allows them to act like weak hormones. Compared with natural estrogens, they are one-thousandth to one-hundred-thousandth as potent. Some experts think that phytoestrogen is not the best name for this group of substances, because it makes it sound like a female hormone and phytoestrogens are beneficial for men, too. But the name is ingrained in both the scientific and the lay literature and it is hard to change it now.

One amazing fact about phytoestrogens is that scientists knew they were present in animals for a very long time before they found them in humans. In the 1940s, sheep in western Australia were having trouble reproducing. When scientists investigated the problem, they learned that those sheep having problems had eaten a type of clover called *Trifolium subterraneum*, which contains a type of isoflavone called equol. You might say the sheep had stumbled upon a plant birth control method.[23] Doctors Messina and Setchell point out that the equol is not actually found in the clover but is converted into this substance by bacteria living in the animal's intestinal tract.[24] Equol sounds a lot like *equus*, the Latin word for horse, because that is the animal in which it was first identified. Before you start worrying that phytoestrogens might affect reproduction in humans, let me reassure you that they do not. But when we include them in our diets, they do have many positive health benefits.

No studies of phytoestrogens in humans existed until 1982.[25] We now know there are two major families of phytoestrogens important to humans—the isoflavones and the lignans. A third group of isoflavones called coumestans are also present in humans but they occur primarily in soy, clover, and alfalfa sprouts so we do not usually eat enough of them to make a major impact.

Soybeans are one of the richest sources of isoflavones, and clover is another fairly rich source. A few other beans besides

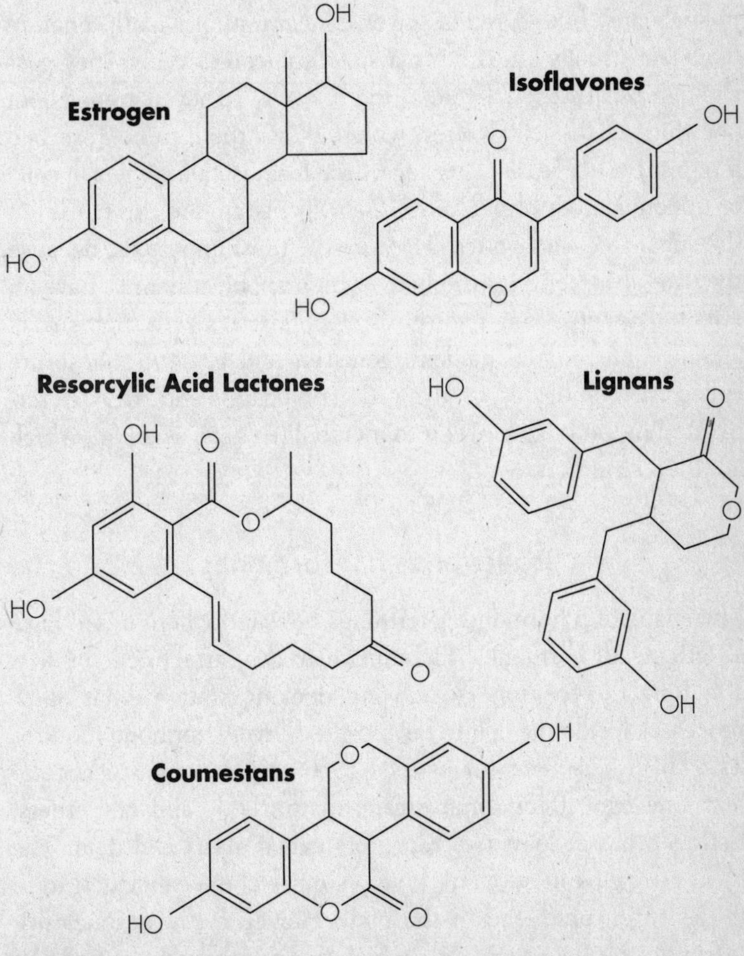

FIGURE 3-3. Chemical Structure of Phytoestrogens

soybeans contain isoflavones, but they are present in much lower concentrations. Flaxseed (linseed) is the richest source of lignans in food, but lignans are also found in some grains such as rye, and in some fruits, vegetables, and berries.

Soy contains two major isoflavones—daidzein and genistein. If you go into a store to buy soy, you will often see these names written on the label. A third isoflavone, glycitein, is also present in soybeans, but in much lower concentrations. Isoflavones in foods are usually attached to a sugar molecule. When they pass through our intestinal tracts, the sugar is removed from about one-third of the isoflavones, which allows them to be absorbed into our bloodstream. This sugar-free form is called the aglycone or unconjugated form. Daidzein and genistein are the names of the sugar-free isoflavones. They are the most important, because they are absorbed into the body, which enables them to have an effect. The remaining two-thirds of isoflavones with their sugars attached are named daidzin, genistin, and glycitin. These are called the conjugated or glycoside conjugates, and they are fermented in the large bowel into metabolites such as equol, which are then absorbed.

Isoflavones as Hormones

The shape of a hormone determines how and where it will have an effect. All hormones, including estrogen, affect cells by first attaching to receptors, which are docking stations that allow processes inside the cell to be activated. Every hormone requires its own unique receptor or receptors. That is why a particular hormone can affect some organs in the body and not others. Estrogen has at least two receptors called alpha and beta. The phytoestrogens in soy have a very similar chemical structure to the estrogen produced in the body. However, soy attaches primarily to the beta receptors, which are mostly prevalent on the bones and cardiovascular system, while estrogen attaches to

TABLE 3-2. ISOFLAVONE CONTENT OF SELECTED FOODS

Food	Isoflavone (mg/100 g food)
Soybeans, green, raw	151.17
Soy flour	148.61
Soy protein isolate	97.43
Soy protein concentrate (alcohol extracted)	12.47
Miso soup, dry	60.39
Tofu (Mori-Nu), silken, firm	31.32
Tofu (Azumaya), extra firm, steamed	22.70
Tofu yogurt	16.30
Soymilk	9.65
Vegetable burgers, prepared (Green Giant Harvest Burgers)	8.22
Soy sauce (from hydrolyzed vegetable protein)	0.10

SOURCE: United States Department of Agriculture. Iowa State University, 1999.

both the beta and alpha receptors, which are primarily on the breasts and uterus. In addition, because phytoestrogens are similar but not identical to human estrogen, they attach to the estrogen receptor but do not cause as strong an effect.

Think of different size airplanes docking at the same terminal gate. Both the larger and the smaller airplane can occupy the same gate. When a small airplane is at the gate, a larger airplane cannot dock there. The site is already occupied. The small plane will have fewer passengers and a much smaller effect on airport traffic. The more small airplanes there are, the less overall impact the larger airplanes can have.

This partial blocking effect of soy may play a protective role for women before menopause when their own estrogen levels are higher. The isoflavones in soy play a protective role, keeping the stronger estrogens that are produced in the body from being able to exert as strong an effect. After menopause, when a woman's own estrogen levels are lower, soy's isoflavones themselves contribute a weak estrogen effect.

Soy and Thyroid

A few studies done on animal cells in culture dishes and in infants given soy-based formulas raise a question whether soy interferes with thyroid function. In Japan, where soy consumption is much higher than in the United States, there is no evidence for increased risk for thyroid disease. Additional proof comes from a randomized, double-blind, placebo-controlled study of 38 menopausal women between the ages of 64 and 83 and not taking hormone replacement. After being given 90 milligrams (mg) of soy isoflavones a day for more than 6 months, no antithyroid evidence was shown.[26] Because thyroid disease is a common problem for menopausal women who may be taking soy, it is easy to see how people might believe one had something to do with the other. There is one note of caution. If you already have thyroid disease and take thyroid hormone, eating soy foods *at the same time* may reduce the amount of thyroid hormone you absorb. If you are worried about your thyroid function, get a simple blood test, and you will know for sure if you have a problem. Meantime, keep taking your soy.

CONCLUSIONS

By now you know about some of the amazing qualities of soy. It is an ancient food possessing great nutritional benefits and

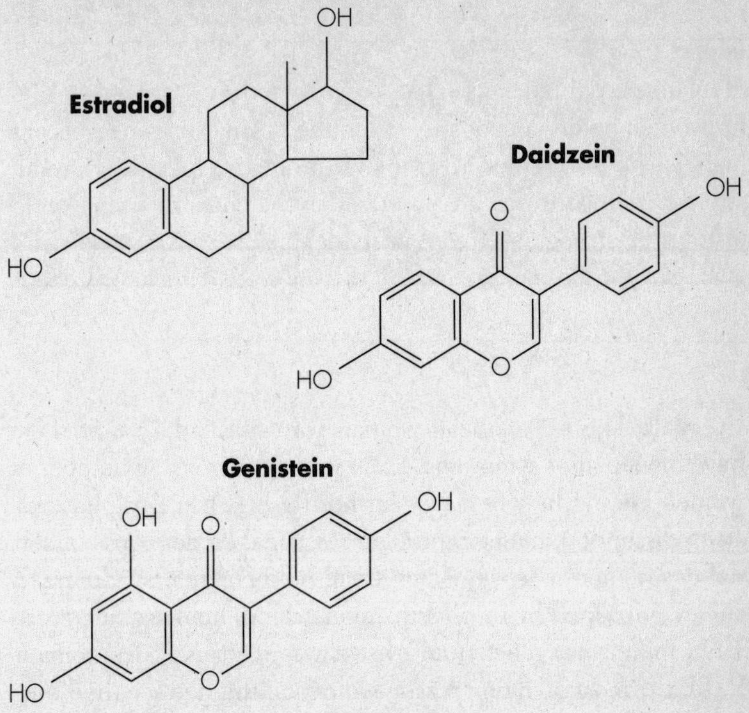

FIGURE 3-4. Estrogen-like Isoflavones

potentially great health benefits. In the following chapters, you will learn how soy can help protect you from the most common conditions that occur in menopause. I believe you will see why I believe that soy is an excellent alternative choice for women approaching and in menopause who either will not or cannot take estrogen.

chapter 4

SOY AND MENOPAUSAL SYMPTOMS

Every day 4,000 American women turn 50, and 75% of them have menopausal symptoms. Each year an increasing number of women ask me how best to treat hot flashes, heart palpitations, sleep disruption, memory problems, vaginal dryness, loss of sexual desire, and a sense of perpetual premenstrual syndrome. A survey published by the North American Menopause Society in 1998 found that relief from everyday menopausal symptoms is by far the most common reason women at this age see their doctors. As Gail Sheehy wrote in *The Silent Passage*, "They feel— and in fact are—out of control of their bodies."[1]

Some women worry that they have a physical illness or have developed a psychological problem. Others have difficulty performing their work or maintaining their relationships at home. All are highly motivated to do something to make themselves feel better and find relief from their symptoms. Women soon learn that estrogen will improve all or most of these symptoms. But what alternative can a doctor offer to women who are unwilling to take estrogen? I believe the single best answer is soy.

HOT FLASHES

"They aren't hot flashes, they're power surges."
Anonymous

In the United States, hot flashes are the most common symptom women associate with menopause. For most women, hot flashes begin when their menstrual cycles become irregular, during the months when they are not menstruating. When their menstrual cycles begin again, the hot flashes stop. But that is not always the case. Some women start having hot flashes while their menstrual cycles are still regular and some do not start having them until several years after menopause has occurred.

The frequency, intensity, and length of hot flashes varies from woman to woman. Most of my patients have occasional hot flashes, but 10% to 15% have them frequently. These women often notice a daily pattern. Many have hot flashes more often and more intensely late in the evening. Intensity and frequency may vary over the course of the day, from day to day, or from season to season. Keep a record of the time and severity of your hot flashes to see if there is a pattern. Dressing and undressing in layers can help you tolerate overheated offices and meeting rooms. At least one study confirms that the frequency and intensity of hot flashes decline dramatically when women are in a cool environment.

Most hot flashes last 3 to 6 minutes, some are shorter, but others can last for more than 30 minutes. How many years you will experience hot flashes can also vary. Some women have them for only about 6 months and others for as long as 40 years. Most have them for 2 or 3 years.

Analysis of a Hot Flash

When you consider what is happening to your body during a hot flash, it is no wonder they have a major impact on the way that you feel. Everyone is different, but most women experience a sudden increase in heart rate that is sensed as palpitations. At the same time, the blood flow to the skin increases, causing your face to flush. Sweating often follows, particularly on the upper body. When the sweat evaporates a few minutes later, the body cools down, and you may feel chilled.

Nobody is sure what sets these events in motion. It is as if the thermostat that regulates a woman's temperature is broken. Hot, humid weather, psychological stress, a confining space, caffeine, alcohol, and spicy foods can trigger hot flashes for some women. When they occur during sleep, there usually is no trigger. According to Dr. Fredi Kronenberg of the College of Physicians and Surgeons at Columbia University in New York City, some women avoid touching, hugging, or sexual activity because the skin-to-skin contact may bring on a hot flash. If you observe the conditions around you at the time of the hot flash, you may be able to exert some control.

Many patients approaching menopause wonder if hot flashes will happen to them. Women who have lower body weight and women who have lower blood levels of estrogen are more likely to have hot flashes. The lower a woman's estrogen level, the more severe her hot flashes. But there is no absolute sign: not how many babies you have had or how old you were when you had your first period, what medical problems you might have had, what type of work you do, your age or marital status, or your employment status.

Why Are Hot Flashes a Problem?

For women who only have them occasionally, hot flashes are not a major problem. But if they are intense enough or happen often enough, hot flashes can be both a source of embarrassment and a disabling and physical drain.

For some women the most upsetting thing about hot flashes is becoming flushed and sweaty in public. Depending on the situation, it can be embarrassing. For the majority of women, the most troublesome problem caused by hot flashes is sleep disturbance. Just as the months and months of getting up at night for a new baby leads to sleep deprivation and chronic tiredness, night-time hot flashes disturb the normal pattern of sleep. It is almost impossible to be sharp and alert when you are exhausted. It is also hard to be calm and understanding with family members under these conditions. Sleep deprivation due to hot flashes plays a major role in creating the anxiety, irritability, and nervousness often associated with menopause.

Soy as an Estrogen Alternative for Hot Flashes

Although as many as 85% of American women and 70% to 80% of European women experience hot flashes, Asian women generally have a different experience. Only 18% of Chinese women, 14% of Singapore women, and an even smaller number of Japanese women complain of this symptom.[2] Why? Most scientists believe it is because of the high levels of soy—which contains phytoestrogens—in their diets. The consumption of soy products is estimated to be highest in some Japanese populations and 5 to 10 times higher throughout Asia than it is in Western countries.

As we learned earlier, the word phytoestrogen literally means plant estrogen, and the type of phytoestrogens found in soy are called isoflavones; the names of the two most abundant isoflavones in soy are genistein and daidzein. Soy is one of the most abundant sources of isoflavones in nature. Isoflavones look very similar to the human female sex hormone estrogen. It has also long been recognized that phytoestrogens exert hormonal effects in cell culture systems and animals. But understanding how soy fits into this simple statement has been confusing, because soy acts differently in premenopausal and post-menopausal women.

As I explained in Chapter 3, soy affects premenopausal and postmenopausal women differently. Estrogen has at least two receptors, called alpha and beta. The phytoestrogens in soy have a very similar chemical structure to the estrogen produced in the body. Because phytoestrogens are similar but not identical to the body's estrogen, they primarily attach to the beta estrogen receptor but do not cause as strong an effect. Estrogen levels are high in premenopausal women. When phytoestrogens attach to the estrogen receptors they prevent the body's stronger estrogen from attaching. It is why soy appears to act as an antiestrogen in premenopausal women. In postmenopausal women the reverse is true and it works like a weak estrogen. The body's estrogen levels are low and soy acts as a weak estrogen because even though it is not as strong, there are very few "large planes" (estrogen) available to attach to the estrogen receptors.

Although it has been known for centuries that few menopausal women in Japan complain of hot flashes, the first scientific evidence that this fact was due to soy consumption was not published until 1992 by some pioneers in soy research.[3] They measured the level of the isoflavones genistein and daidzein in the urine of menopausal Japanese, American, and Finnish women. They found 100 times more excretion in the urine of the Japanese women compared with American and Finnish women. The level of urinary phytoestrogens reflects how much soy the person has eaten—the more one eats, the higher the level of phytoestrogens in the urine. Women who consume large amounts of soy have higher urine values of phytoestrogens than those who consume smaller quantities. The excretion of isoflavones in the urine was associated with the intake of a variety of soy products, such as tofu, miso, aburage, atuage, kori-dofu, soybeans, and boiled beans. In fact, Japanese women eat so much soy that the level of phytoestrogens excreted in their urine is 100 to 1,000 times higher than the level of their own body's estrogens. These striking differences in phytoestrogen levels are the basis for the efficacy of soy in reducing hot flashes and other menopausal symptoms. Even though phytoestrogens are "weak" estrogens, their high concentration makes them bio-logically important.

Other important studies followed. Murkies and colleagues studied 58 menopausal women suffering from hot flashes and supplemented their diets with 45 grams of soy flour daily.[4] A comparison group received the same amount of bleached wheat, which contained virtually no isoflavones. By 12 weeks, the women who received soy flour had 40% fewer hot flashes daily. The comparison group also improved, but only by 25%.

Another study of 145 menopausal women used a dietitian to educate the participants.[5] Half the women were told how to avoid phytoestrogens and the other half were told how to supple-ment their diet with approximately one fourth of their caloric intake from phytoestrogens (mostly soy but also some flaxseed). As in the first study, both groups found their menopausal symp-toms improved, but the women consuming phytoestrogens improved significantly more.

An Italian group also studied the effects of soy supplementa-tion on hot flashes.[6] Fifty-one patients aged 48 to 61 took 60 grams of soy protein daily, and 53 similarly aged patients took a placebo. Both groups experienced some improvement but soy was significantly superior to the placebo in reducing the number of daily hot flashes. Women taking soy had a 26% reduction by 3 weeks, a 33% reduction by week 4, and a 45% reduction in the mean number of hot flashes by the end of week 12, versus a 30% reduction with the placebo.

In January 2001, a group of Japanese doctors published a study on the benefits of soy on Japanese postmenopausal women.[7] They divided the 478 women into two groups—those who had gone through menopause less than 5 years ago (early group) and those who had gone through it more than 5 years ago (late group). They also looked at how much soy these women actually ate. Of course, all of the women were eating some soy, but some ate more and some ate less. The results were very interesting. Japanese women who ate more soy (food containing 65 milligrams [mg] per day of isoflavones) had less menopausal symptoms than those eating smaller amounts. The benefits were greatest early in menopause because that is when symptoms tend to be most noticeable. Higher soy intake was particularly helpful in reducing the amount of palpitations and backache the women experienced.

All of these studies have found similar results—soy is able to significantly reduce menopausal symptoms. Even in Japan where everyone eats soy, those who eat a little more soy tend to have fewer menopausal symptoms.

Soy Supplements Versus Soy Food

Whenever there is discussion of using plants for their medicinal benefits, a discussion usually follows as to whether using a pill or tablet that contains important ingredients found in the plant is comparable to eating the plant. Certainly, this question comes up all the time in the nutritional supplement industry where $46 billion of vitamins, minerals, herbs, and other nutritional supplements are sold each year throughout the world. Not only is it a fair question, it is also an important one, because the answer for each nutritional supplement must be considered individually rather than about the industry as a whole.

I became particularly interested in this question regarding soy in the mid-1990s. At the time, I had been in practice roughly 20 years. More and more of my patients were entering menopause, and like women of similar age across the United States, many did not want to take estrogen. I found myself talking more about soy, offering recipes, and discussing other ways of including soy into my patients' diets. Obviously, this was not the usual discussion at a gynecologist's annual examination. Many of my patients took my advice, but did not eat soy every day, which would be the ideal way to get the most from soy's potential benefits. Others could not get used to the taste. I started wondering if a soy supplement for hot flashes would work. I knew it would be easier for many women to take.

About that time I was approached by Inverness Medical, Inc., a publicly traded company, to consult with them about developing a soy supplement that could be used to help cope with hot flashes. I found myself walking through organic soy fields in this country's heartland, touring enormous processing plants where acres of soybeans are processed each hour, and gaining a great understanding of soy isoflavones.

The end result was the development of SoyCare Menopause—one of the first nutritional supplements intended to help women reduce their hot flashes. All of the soy ingredients are organically grown, not genetically modified (GMO free), and each capsule contains 25 mg of isoflavones. One capsule, taken twice daily, keeps the blood levels of the isoflavones in the same range throughout the day, which mimics people eating a typical Asian diet. I felt this was important, since people who eat soy usually consume it in more than one meal daily. I also insisted that if women were not satisfied, they could get their money back for the product. Lest this sound like a promotion, I do not make any money from the sales of SoyCare. But I am able to reach a lot more women than I ever could by sitting in my office.

Since the development of SoyCare, other soy supplements have come on the market, including Healthy Woman and Caltrate 600 Plus Soy.

Several studies using soy isoflavone supplements to treat hot flashes have been conducted in the past few years. In one study, participants in the control group were given a placebo while the treatment group received a supplement containing 50 mg of isoflavones per day.[8] After 6 weeks of treatment, the soy group

TABLE 4-1. COMPARISON OF MAJOR SOY SUPPLEMENTS

Brand	Organic Soy	GMO Free	mg/ Capsule	Dosages/ Day
SoyCare Menopause	Yes	Yes	25	2
Healthy Woman	No	No	50	1
Caltrate 600 Plus Soy	No	No	50	1

had a significant reduction (45%) in hot flashes and night sweats compared with the placebo group (25%). Another recent group of investigators used 50 mg of isoflavones in a double-blind, randomized, placebo-controlled study in 177 patients and confirmed the benefits of soy supplements on hot flashes.[9] Soy isoflavone extract was effective in reducing the frequency and severity of hot flashes and did not cause the uterine lining to have any effects typically seen with estrogen. Eating the entire soybean is ideal, but soy supplements also reduce hot flashes for women who do not eat soy foods regularly.

Interpreting the Data

Some people have been skeptical about the ability of soy to reduce hot flashes. They agree that soy is effective and works better than the placebo, but they also comment that the placebo seems to be quite effective as well. The skeptics ask, if soy is only 15% to 20% better than placebo, even though that is statistically significant, is it meaningful?

The answer is an overwhelming "Yes!" Here is why. So far, all the clinical studies about soy and hot flashes have tested women for no more than 12 weeks. Twenty-year-old studies comparing prescription estrogen to placebo found the same type of results. For 3 months, women taking estrogen showed significant improvement in their hot flashes, but the placebo group also showed some improved symptoms. After 3 months, however, the placebo effect stopped working and the hot flashes became worse for the placebo group but not for the estrogen group. Longer studies were needed to show clearly that estrogen was better than a placebo for reducing hot flashes.[10]

In the meantime, there is another important reason that taking soy makes a difference for women who are suffering from hot flashes. It is true that most women's hot flashes will not go away entirely while taking soy. But it is equally true that soy will usually significantly reduce their hot flashes. Research shows that hot flashes destroy the quality of sleep in peri- and post-menopausal women by affecting rapid eye movement (REM) sleep.[11] It makes sense. How can anyone feel rested in the morning if they are awakened repeatedly throughout the night?

When soy significantly reduces the frequency and severity of hot flashes, it improves the quality of sleep. That may be enough to accomplish what women taking soy already know: Soy can improve the quality of life sufficiently to allow them to get by without taking estrogen.

Put my own way:

ODE TO SOY AND HOT FLASHES

Drenched with sweat I wake again
'Cause I'm afraid of estrogen
Can't recall how long it's been
Since I could sleep the night.

Trying soy could do no harm
It stopped the heat, though I'm still warm.
Now I feel my life is charmed
'Cause I can sleep the night.

Experts say, "It's not the same
As estrogen," they all complain.
But it sure helped turn down the flame.
And I can sleep the night!

VAGINAL DRYNESS AND MENOPAUSE

Vaginal dryness that causes an almost constant soreness or burning and makes intercourse extremely painful is another major symptom of menopause. It is caused by thinning of the vaginal walls due to lower levels of estrogen. Vaginal dryness may affect 80% of women at one time or another. In a survey conducted by *Consumer Reports* magazine, more than half of its female readers used over-the-counter lubricants to reduce unpleasant friction during intercourse. Vaginal dryness is a major reason women seek treatment.

In a survey of patients in private gynecologic practices, few women described experiencing sexual dysfunction, but many admitted to sexual dysfunction when they were presented with a sample of vaginal lubricant.[12] Others do not complain of sexual dysfunction per se, but complain that their partners have become "too quick" or "too uncaring of their needs." The makers of one brand of vaginal lubrication ask, "Are your patients ready for the Viagra revolution?" Vaginal dryness is a major menopausal symptom. Adding soy to the diet is one simple treatment for this problem.

What Causes the Problem?

The cells that line the vagina are sensitive markers of how much estrogen is in the body. In premenopausal women, estrogen levels are higher and the vaginal cells multiply and take on a characteristic appearance that is easily recognized under a microscope. During a physical examination, the walls of the vagina look pinker, thicker, and corrugated. In postmenopausal women, estrogen levels are lower, the number of vaginal cells are less numerous, and each cell takes on a different but also distinct look, and the walls of the vagina are paler, thinner, and flatter.

When a postmenopausal woman receives estrogen, the vaginal cells change back to their estrogenized appearance, and the woman will feel the difference during intercourse. If a menopausal woman develops atrophic vaginitis, a common vaginal inflammation related to low levels of estrogen, it too will clear up if estrogen is given.

The Evidence for Soy

Several studies have been performed using soy to treat vaginal dryness. In one, a group of postmenopausal women not taking estrogen were given equivalent amounts of either soy flour (45 grams daily), red clover sprouts (another source of isoflavones, 10 grams of dry seed daily), or linseed (25 grams daily) to see what effect it had on their vaginal cells. After 6 weeks, the women taking soy and linseed (but not red clover) had noticeable changes in their vaginal cells. When the soy or linseed was discontinued, the changes continued for another 2 weeks and then returned to their baseline appearance.[13]

The study by Brzezinski and colleagues mentioned earlier also looked at the role of phytoestrogens on vaginal dryness. They found that vaginal dryness was significantly improved in women eating a phytoestrogen-enriched diet. Although the information is clouded, because the women in this study were eating 2 teaspoons of ground flaxseed in addition to soy, the authors add a little more evidence to support the role of soy in helping with this problem.

While not every study of soy has shown it to be effective, the fact that some do makes soy a reasonable choice to try for vaginal dryness. Table 4-2 summarizes the available studies.

TABLE 4-2. SOY'S EFFECT ON VAGINAL DRYNESS

Number in Study	Type of Soy	Amount	Effect	Author
25	Soy flour	45 g	Yes	Wilcox
58	Soy flour	45 g	No	Murkies
97	Textured vegetable protein	⅓ calories	No	Baird
52	Soy grits	45 g	Yes	Dalais
145	Tofu + flax	¼ calories	Yes	Brzezinski

THE BOTTOM LINE

Menopausal symptoms are the main reason women see their doctors for help. Most physicians will suggest estrogen as a way to treat them. You will get relief if you take their suggestion. But you can also improve your symptoms without an office visit if you simply incorporate soy or soy supplements into your diet.

chapter 5

SOY AND OSTEOPOROSIS

The doctor of the future will give us no medicine, but will interest his patients in the care of the human frame, in diet and in the cause and prevention of disease.

Thomas Edison

Did you know that the United States is rated along with Scandinavia and central Europe as having the highest per capita incidence of hip fractures in the world? Did you realize that a 50-year-old Caucasian postmenopausal woman has the exact same risk of dying from an osteoporosis-related hip fracture as she does from breast cancer? That she has a four times higher risk of dying from an osteoporosis-related hip fracture as she does from uterine cancer?[1] Osteoporosis is one of the most important diseases facing this country. Many of my patients believe it will not affect them. They are too young or too healthy. They may be very wrong.

Osteoporosis is a silent epidemic that affects millions of unsuspecting women. It is an equal opportunity disease that can afflict the young and the old. Here are three examples of patients I have seen recently:

- Julia is a 35-year-old black woman in excellent health with no medical complaints. On her first visit she told me that she went through menopause when she was only 25 years old.

She does not take any medications. Because of her premature menopause (before age 40), which lowered her estrogen
levels at an early age, I recommended she have a bone-density test. The results showed severe osteoporosis.

- Ann is 45 years old and white. She is the perfect weight for
her 5-foot 5-inch frame and she keeps in shape by combining
an excellent diet with regular walking. She has not gone
through menopause, but she has noticed that her periods are
a little lighter, suggesting menopause might be approaching.
For that reason I recommended she have a bone-density test.
To her amazement, Ann had significant bone loss approaching osteoporosis.

- Janet is 55 years old and went through menopause 4 years ago.
She tried taking estrogen briefly but stopped because of side
effects. Except for the fact that she is slightly overweight and
has mild asthma, she has been healthy until 2 years ago when
her asthma became severe. Janet's internist prescribed a high
dosage of steroids to help control her asthma. When she came
in recently for a yearly exam her life had changed. She developed pain in her left hip that could not be explained until a
magnetic resonance imaging (MRI) test found a fracture of
her left hipbone. A few months later she developed pain in her
right ankle that an X-ray showed to be another fracture. Just
one week before she came in for her exam she was pulling up
her pantyhose and broke her right index finger. "I'm falling
apart," she told me in tears. "My bones just won't hold me up."
Because of her age and history, and the fact that she was taking steroids, Janet agreed to have a bone-density test. I'm sure
by now you have guessed she had significant osteoporosis.

BONES—A LIVING TISSUE

When we think of living tissue, a beating heart is an active type
of image that often comes to mind. Bones, on the other hand,

seem inactive, like Halloween skeletons. That could not be further from the truth. Healthy bones are active living tissue, allowing us to grow when we are younger and permitting our bones to mend if they break.

In fact, bones are constantly active, repairing small defects by a process called bone remodeling. The process starts on the bone's surface in nearly 2 million places at any one time. Special bone cells called osteoclasts remove discrete packets of old bone. This process is called resorption. Once the small crack or rough area is nibbled away, osteoblast cells move into and line the area, filling it with an equal amount of new bone. It takes the body about 10 days to nibble out the old bone and about 90 days to replace it. Throughout life this very active process continues. Calcium constantly is taken out of bones and constantly being replaced. As long as the flow of calcium into and out of bones occurs at the same rate, bone health is maintained.

KEEPING CALCIUM BLOOD LEVELS CONSTANT

Bone remodeling also allows our bones to serve as a reservoir for calcium. About 99% of the 3 pounds of calcium we carry around with us is in our bones. The other 1% of calcium is in our bloodstream and is used for a variety of vital functions, such as keeping our heart beating properly, our blood clotting, or signals traveling down our nerves. The body must keep calcium blood levels in a narrow range because blood levels of calcium that are either too high or too low can be life threatening.

Two hormones help keep this process in balance: parathyroid hormone (PTH) and calcitonin. The parathyroid glands are four tiny glands that sit in front of the thyroid gland, which is located in the neck. Parathyroid hormone increases bone resorption, which takes calcium out of bones. Calcitonin is secreted by the C-cells within the thyroid gland. Calcitonin helps put calcium back into bones and slows down the process of resorption.

If we do not get enough calcium in our diet, especially after menopause, calcium blood levels drop. That signals PTH to increase bone resorption and shift calcium from our bones into our bloodstream. If this happens over a long period of time, the bones become porous. Hence the term osteoporosis or porous bones. The denser our bones are to begin with, the longer it takes for osteoporosis to occur.

MEDICAL HISTORY THAT INCREASES OSTEOPOROSIS RISK

- Anorexia
- Removal of the ovaries or premature menopause (before age 40)
- Lactose intolerance
- Certain prescription and over-the-counter drugs
- Extended bed rest or immobilization
- Removal of part of the stomach or small intestines or problems absorbing food
- Eating disorders, chronic diarrhea, and kidney or liver disease
- Severe hot flashes, especially if lasting 15-plus years

Your medical history can provide clues that suggest an increased risk for developing osteoporosis. Medications such as steroids, anticonvulsants, excessive thyroid medication, and the blood thinner heparin all increase bone loss. So do smoking and excessive alcohol and caffeine consumption.[2] If you are a small, thin, white female with a family history of osteoporosis, your risk of developing osteoporosis is even higher.

HOW BIG IS THE PROBLEM?

Osteoporosis affects approximately 28 million Americans, and 80% of them are women. As a result of this disease, 16% of women over the age of 50 will break their hips and nearly 33% will fracture and compress their backbones causing a loss of height. Nearly half of all women over 50 will have some type of bone fracture due to osteoporosis. A person who has one bone fracture is 2 to 5 times more likely to have another. The sites of these fractures are the spine (650,000), the hip (250,000), the forearm (200,000), and other skeletal sites (400,000).[3] The annual health-care costs due to osteoporosis are almost $14 billion, and this number is expected to reach $60 billion over the next 20 years, largely because of the enormous numbers of aging baby boomers.[4]

The personal cost may be even higher. If a woman breaks her hip after age 70, she will have a 20% chance of dying within the following year. Half the survivors will lose their independence, because they will not be able to walk unassisted, and 25% will be confined to long-term care in a nursing home. Listening to my patients' comments, fear of losing their independence and looking disfigured due to a dowager's hump may be the most frightening aspects of osteoporosis. Fortunately, the risk of developing osteoporosis can be greatly reduced if people seek treatment early. According to the American Medical Association, the following are symptoms to look out for:

WARNING SIGNS OF OSTEOPOROSIS

- Chronic low back pain
- Loss of height
- Breaking a hip with minimal trauma or any other bone with no trauma
- Leg cramps at night
- Joint pain
- Tooth loss
- Periodontal (gum) disease

TEETH ARE BONES, TOO

When most people think about bones they usually don't think of teeth. But the teeth can also be affected by osteoporosis. Studies suggest that by age 60, up to 40% of otherwise healthy women will have lost all their teeth.[5] Part of the reason is that the jawbone in which teeth are planted is made of trabecular bone, a type that is more porous to begin with than the compact long bones of the arms and legs. The rate of bone loss speeds up at the time of menopause and now a formula for tooth loss is in place.

DIAGNOSING OSTEOPOROSIS

Even though there are many warning signs, the majority of women with osteoporosis have no clinical sign or symptom.[6] That is why I think that every woman age 40, and definitely by age 50, should have a screening bone-density exam. If there is a strong medical history or warning signs, it should be even earlier. To me it is just as important a screening tool as a mammogram because a 50-year-old white postmenopausal woman has the identical risk of one day dying from a fracture related to osteoporosis as she does dying from breast cancer.

Some bone-density tests use sound waves (ultrasound), but most use low X-ray doses similar to the sun's radiation exposure during air travel. The test measures the density of a woman's bones and compares it to women of the same age (Z-score) and to young women at the peak of their bone density (T-score). Osteoporosis is defined as 2.5 standard deviations or greater below the mean. For each standard deviation reduction in T-score, the risk of eventually having a fracture related to osteoporosis increases by a whopping 50%.[7] I believe that measurements of the hip are the most accurate, followed by the spine, but newer machines measuring bone density in the heel, wrist, forearm, kneecap, and fingers also are useful for screening osteoporosis.[8] Whichever technology you use, it is important to realize that a T-score at the same site by a different technology is not equivalent. The different technologies are not standardized.[9]

Biochemical tests for bone loss in blood and urine are also available. They measure specific proteins, C- and N-terminal telopeptides, that increase when there is increased bone resorption.[10] If this test is elevated, get a bone-density exam. People being treated for osteoporosis can also use this test—bone resorption slows down if treatment is working. Soy also helps slow resorption.

FOR BEST PREVENTION, START YOUNG

The first 10 years of the new millennium will see the U.S. teenage population grow in number at almost twice the rate of the general population, exceeding 30 million by the year 2015 and exceeding the number of teenagers created by the baby boomers in the 1960s and 1970s.[11] It is during adolescence and young adulthood that young women have the lowest intake of calcium—less than 60% of the recommended daily allowance. Unfortunately, this is exactly the time when the body is using calcium to build strong bones. By the age of 17, 91% of a woman's ultimate bone mass is built and most of the remaining 9% is built by the mid-20s. By 30, the goal is simply to hold on to the level that has been achieved.[12]

The poor intake of calcium by teenagers was highlighted in a study of mothers and their daughters. The mothers, whose average age was 44, had not yet reached menopause. Their daughters' average age was 18. The mothers were found to have about 10% more calcium in their bones than their daughters.[13] If one assumes that mothers and daughters will lose bone at the same rate because they are genetically similar, diet must play a significant role. The bottom line is, one of the best ways to lower the likelihood of developing osteoporosis in future generations of menopausal women is to start working on the problem in child-hood and young adult life.

MENOPAUSE SPEEDS BONE LOSS

Bones are thickest when a woman is in her mid- to late 20s. After that, bone is slowly lost. About one fourth of the total amount of bone is lost before menopause. After menopause, bone loss speeds up. Another 10% will be lost from the long bones of the body, and another 25% will be lost from the spine and hips. All together, this amounts to 35% of the long bones of the body and half of the spine and pelvis. This is why it is so important in youth to build as much bone as possible and to slow down the rate of loss before, during, and after menopause.

The good news is it is never too late. Researchers from France reported in the *New England Journal of Medicine* that vitamin D and calcium (in the form of calcium triphosphate) reduced the risk of hip fracture in a group of women more than 70 years of age by 43% over an 18-month study.[14] As blood levels of calcium increased, their release of PTH slowed down, and with it, so did the number of hip fractures. The only calcium supplement widely sold in the United States that contains calcium triphosphate and vitamin D is Posture D.

DIET AND OSTEOPOROSIS

Food choices and dietary habits play a large role in bone health. One cup of low-fat milk contains 300 milligrams (mg) of calcium; an ounce of mozzarella cheese, about 200 mg. Dairy products are not the only foods rich in calcium. A half cup of dry roasted soybeans contains 232 mg of calcium and one-fourth block of tofu contains from 166 mg up to 553 mg if calcium sulfate is used as the curdling agent rather than nigari, the traditional curdling agent found in natural sea salt.

Obtaining a portion of dietary calcium from vegetable sources is wise for two reasons. One has to do with the high fat content in many of the calcium-rich sources of dairy products. Too much fat in the diet can contribute to an increased risk of heart disease. The second reason is the large amount of animal protein present in dairy foods. For each gram of protein consumed, 1 mg of calcium is lost in the urine. Protein increases the acid load of urine and requires calcium to be used as a buffer.[15] This point is seldom considered in discussions of the popular high-protein diets.

Even the type of protein can make a difference. People who get their protein from meat and dairy foods lose 50% more calcium from their bodies than people who eat only soy protein. Too much sodium can also cause calcium to be lost in the urine. For every gram of sodium eaten, loss of calcium from the urine increases by 26 mg. It is easy to understand how a diet that consists largely of sodas, hamburgers, and salty French fries might contribute to osteoporosis. It may turn out that for many American women, osteoporosis is not caused by too little calcium in the diet, but rather too much animal protein and salt causing excessive calcium loss.

BONING UP ON CALCIUM

Doctors have learned that getting enough calcium intake reduces bone loss and the risk of osteoporosis in menopausal women by approximately 0.8% per year. That is 40% better than it would be if too little calcium were consumed. This information led the Institute of Medicine of the National Academy of Sciences to recommend that healthy women who are older than 50 should consume 1,200 mg of calcium daily rather than the 800 mg per day recommended earlier.[16] Even so, postmenopausal women in the United States only get on average 563 mg per day of calcium from their diet, less than half the recommended amount. Those

TABLE 5-1. CALCIUM, CALORIE, AND FAT CONTENT OF COMMON DAIRY FOODS

	Calcium (mg)	Calories	Fat (g)
Milk and milk beverages			
Milk, whole, 1 cup	291	150	8
Milk, low fat (2%), 1 cup	297	120	5
Milk, low fat (1%), 1 cup	300	100	1
Milk, skim, 1 cup	302	85	0
Chocolate milk, (1%), 1 cup	287	160	1
Buttermilk, 1 cup	285	100	2
Cheeses			
American, 1 oz	174	105	9
Cheddar, 1 oz	204	115	9
Cottage, low fat (1%), 1 cup	155	160	2
Mozzarella, part skim, 1 oz	207	80	5
Swiss, 1 oz	272	105	8
Yogurt			
Plain, low fat, 8 oz	415	145	3
Plain, nonfat, 8 oz	452	125	0
Fruit, low fat, 8 oz	345	230	3
Coffee or vanilla, 8 oz	389	194	3
Desserts			
Ice milk, hardened, 1 cup	176	185	6
Ice milk, soft serve, 1 cup	274	225	5
Ice cream (11% milk fat), 1 cup	176	270	14
Sherbet (2% fat), 1 cup	103	270	6
Other Good Sources of Calcium			
Almonds	75	165	16
Broccoli, cooked, ½ cup	47	25	0
Collard greens, cooked, ½ cup	179	30	0
Kale, cooked, ½ cup	90	20	0
Salmon, pink, canned, with liquid and bones, 3 oz	167	120	5
Sardines, canned in oil, with liquid and bones, 3 oz	371	175	9
Snap beans, cooked, ½ cup	31	18	0
Tofu, firm, raw, ¼ block	166	118	7.1
Curdled with calcium salt	553	118	7.1

(continued)

TABLE 5-1. CALCIUM, CALORIE, AND FAT CONTENT OF COMMON DAIRY FOODS (continued)

	Calcium (mg)	Calories	Fat (g)
Tofu, regular, raw, ¼ block	122	88	5.6
Curdled with calcium salt	406	88	5.6
Soybeans, dry roasted, ½ cup	232	387	18.6
Soybeans, boiled, ½ cup	88	149	7.7
Soy protein concentrate, 1 oz	102	93	0.13

SOURCE: Modified from Seibel MM. The role of nutrition and nutritional supplements in women's health. *Fertil Steril.* 1999;72:579–591.

postmenopausal women need to take a calcium supplement. This has translated into American consumers spending $1 million each day ($365 million annually) for calcium supplements.

Calcium also improves the ability of estrogen to prevent osteoporosis. When estrogen is taken alone, the bone mass of the lower spine increases 1.3% per year compared with 3.3% per year when calcium is given along with the estrogen. The femoral neck, which is the upper part of the thigh bone that connects it to the hip, also increases in bone density when calcium is given with estrogen, from 0.9% per year to 2.4%.[17] These positive results have caused some physicians to recommend to their patients who already have osteoporosis to take even more than

TABLE 5-2. RECOMMENDED DAILY CALCIUM INTAKE

4- to 8-year-olds	1,000 mg/day
9- to 18-year-olds	1,550 mg/day
Pregnant/breast feeding adult	1,200 mg/day
Premenopausal adult	1,000 mg/day
Postmenopausal adult	
Taking estrogen	1,000 mg/day
Not taking estrogen	1,500 mg/day

SOURCE: National Academy of Science.

the recommended amounts—up to 2,000 mg per day. Higher dosages of calcium do have a potential downside. They can cause kidney stones. Drinking 8 to 12 glasses of water daily, especially in hot climates, minimizes this risk.

Factors Affecting Calcium Absorption

Understanding calcium absorption can be tricky. Not only does it depend on calcium per se, but also on other factors. For instance, taking too much calcium at once actually lowers the efficiency of its absorption. A plateau is reached at a dose of about 500 to 600 mg.[18] That is why it makes sense to take calcium supplements in divided doses rather than taking them all at once. Taking a second calcium tablet before bedtime may also reduce calcium loss from bones during the night.[19]

Certain foods and nutrients also affect calcium absorption. In general, it is better to take a calcium supplement with meals, because eating increases the stomach's acidity, which helps the absorption of calcium. But, according to Mark Twain, "All generalizations are inaccurate, including this one." Eating a meal that contains carbohydrates increases the absorption of calcium. Soy is an excellent source of calcium and may even increase the amount of calcium that our bodies can absorb from food.[20] But soy protein taken together with a calcium supplement will bind the calcium and reduce the amount absorbed. The same is true for wheat bran.

Soy isoflavones found in supplements and sometimes combined with calcium do not reduce calcium absorption. Neither does the fiber in green, leafy vegetables and in psyllium. Other foods such as spinach and rhubarb have high concentrations of calcium, but almost none of the calcium is absorbed because they also contain high concentrations of oxalic acid.[21, 22] In contrast, calcium supplements interfere with the absorption of iron. People who need to take both calcium and iron supplements should not take them at the same time. The more aware you are of these types of interactions, the more effectively you can plan what you eat, and the more capable your body will be to use the calcium you consume.

Calcium Supplements

Calcium supplements represent nearly two thirds of all the mineral supplements sold. There are dozens of different preparations available over the counter. Customers purchase roughly $1 million worth of them each day. Calcium is sold as a "salt," which means the calcium is attached to another substance— usually carbonate, citrate, or phosphate. Each of these salts contains different percentages of calcium.

When food enters the stomach, acid is secreted to aid in digestion. The acid also helps dissolve calcium supplements. So take yours with food.

TABLE 5-3. CALCIUM CONTENT OF VARIOUS CALCIUM "SALTS"

Type of Calcium	% Calcium
Carbonate	40
Tricalcium phosphate	38
Dicalcium phosphate	31
Bone meal	31
Oyster shell	28
Dolomite	22
Citrate	21
Lactate	13
Gluconate (mostly given intravenously)	9
Glubionate (mostly in syrups for kids)	6.5

SOURCE: Levenson DI, Bockman RS. A review of calcium preparations. *Nutr Rev.* 1994;52:221–232.

Calcium carbonate is the most commonly used calcium salt because it is the least expensive. It can be made from chalk or calcium hydroxide and occurs naturally in limestone and oyster shell. Calcium carbonate is poorly absorbed on an empty stomach. Tums antacid, a popular form of calcium carbonate, is even less well absorbed because antacids neutralize the stomach's acidity. Many people also complain that it tastes like chalk. Taken with meals, calcium carbonate's absorption improves considerably.

Calcium citrate is sold both as a tablet and as an effervescent preparation. It is better absorbed on an empty stomach than calcium carbonate, but because it contains less calcium by weight, it takes nearly twice as many tablets to get the same amount of calcium as it does if either calcium carbonate or calcium phosphate are taken.

Calcium phosphate (as tribasic phosphate), available in 600-mg tablets taken twice daily, may cause less gas distress and less constipation than other calcium salts.[23] As with calcium carbonate, it is best absorbed with food.

Two natural sources of calcium, dolomite and bone meal, deserve special mention. Dolomite is a natural mineral combination of calcium carbonate and magnesium carbonate, both of which can contain low levels of lead and other toxic metals.[24] Bone meal is usually made from ground-up cow bones. It is poorly absorbed and tastes bad. Although purely hypothetical, the possibility for getting mad cow disease or other diseases from cows' ground-up bone marrow makes it an unacceptable choice for me. Bone meal may also contain relatively high levels of lead.[25] Dolomite and bone meal are two examples where natural is not better.

PHOSPHOROUS—THE FORGOTTEN NUTRIENT

Almost everyone knows that calcium is necessary for healthy bones. Less people are aware that bone health also requires phosphorous. Although many women get enough phosphorous from their diet, 50 million women have dietary intakes of phosphorous below the daily recommended levels. (U.S. Census Bureau, December 2000.) According to Dr. Robert P. Heaney of Creighton University in Omaha, Nebraska, an expert in bone metabolism, when women with low or low normal phosphorous levels take calcium as a supplement, it can actually lower their phosphorous levels even more. Calcium binds phosphorous in the intestinal tract and prevents this essential element from being absorbed. For this reason, choosing the wrong calcium supplement could actually make the risk for osteoporosis worse. Dr. Heaney reported on March 9, 2002 at the Fifth International Symposium: Clinical Advances in Osteoporosis that calcium phosphate was the safest calcium supplement to help our patients meet their needs for both calcium and phosphorous. As stated earlier, the only major calcium phosphate supplement on the market is Posture D.

VITAMIN D—AN ESSENTIAL VITAMIN FOR BONE HEALTH

Vitamin D is an important ingredient in bone health. Without it the body cannot absorb calcium from the intestinal tract, and even eating calcium or taking a calcium supplement will not improve bone density. If our blood levels of calcium become too low, vitamin D also helps to remove calcium from the bones and bring it into the bloodstream. It helps the kidneys reabsorb calcium, so it is not lost in the urine. Vitamin D may also play a role in reducing the risk of certain cancers.[26]

Children are born with enough vitamin D to last them nine months. After that it has to be eaten or manufactured by the body. Vitamin D comes in one of three forms—calciferol, cholecalciferol, and ergocalciferol. Calciferol is naturally occurring in fish oils and egg yolk. It is the type of vitamin D that is added to margarine and milk in the United States. The body manufactures cholecalciferol if it is exposed to about 15 minutes of sunlight daily. Sunlight activates a compound in the body fat beneath the skin. It is stored in the liver until needed and is then converted in the kidneys to an active form of vitamin D. The ability of sunlight to make vitamin D is reduced by sunscreen, smog, and clothing that covers all the skin. Ergocalciferol is synthesized in plants when they are exposed to sunlight.

After menopause, the body becomes less capable of manufacturing vitamin D from exposure to sunlight. Women who live in more northern climates where exposure to sunlight is short during the winter months or who are confined inside need more vitamin D. So do obese people, because it deposits itself in the body's fat and does not make itself available in the bloodstream.[27] To be certain there is enough vitamin D, either eat more foods containing vitamin D or take a supplement that contains it. Foods rich in vitamin D include milk fortified with vitamin D, fortified breakfast cereals, egg yolks, canned sardines, canned tuna, saltwater fish, and liver. The total amount of vitamin D taken from supplements should be between 400 and 800 IU daily. This is equivalent to 10 to 20 micrograms of cholecalciferol.

BALANCING CALCIUM AND MAGNESIUM

In one survey, only 25% of Americans had a dietary intake of magnesium that equaled or exceeded the recommended daily allowance (RDA).[28] Pregnant women in the United States ingest only 35% to 58% of the RDA.[29] For calcium to be incorporated into bones it needs magnesium. Without adequate magnesium, some calcium intended for bones will end up in soft tissues and cause calcium deposits. I am concerned that many women taking calcium supplements but not taking magnesium may be causing some of the benign calcifications that show up frequently on mammograms.

The average person needs about one third to one half as much magnesium as they do calcium. So if you are taking 1,200 mg of calcium daily, you also need 400 to 600 mg of magnesium. Some calcium supplements also contain magnesium, but this may reduce absorption of magnesium in the digestive tract. Magnesium also makes the stomach less acidic, which slows down the absorption of food. For best results, take a separate magnesium supplement at a separate time. This is true even if your entire source of calcium is from dairy products because dairy products contain nine times more calcium than they do magnesium. Foods rich in magnesium are leafy green vegetables, nuts, seeds, sea vegetables, and soy, particularly soybeans and tofu. Almonds are particularly rich in magnesium, containing 120 mg per one-fourth cup. Chinese, Indian, and other Oriental foods are also good sources. Sugar and alcohol cause magnesium loss by the kidneys.

About the only common side effect of magnesium is diarrhea. It is more likely with inorganic forms (magnesium oxide, magnesium chloride) than it is with organic forms (magnesium citrate, magnesium aspartate), but diarrhea can occur with any preparation.[30]

NOT EVERYBODY CAN DRINK MILK

Most of the information bandied about concerning bone health has to do with calcium and vitamin D. But as we have already learned, understanding bone health is complicated. Ann Louise Gittleman in her book *Before the Change* makes the point that our bodies do not differ much from our Stone Age ancestors 40,000 years ago. However, our diets do. Because animals have only been domesticated for 10,000 years, milk and milk products are a relatively new food. Before that time, the only milk available was mother's milk.

That is probably why so many people over 4 years old are at least somewhat lactose intolerant. Lactose is the sugar found in milk. Our intestines break it down with the help of the enzyme lactase. After age 4 many people's intestines stop making lactase, so they cannot digest lactose. When it enters the intestine, bacteria ferment the lactose, causing gas, bloating, cramps, and sometimes, diarrhea. People of African, Native American, Greek, Arab, Ashkenazi or Sephardic Jewish, or Oriental ancestry are more likely to have this condition. Soy is a wonderful alternative to milk and milk products—a rich source of calcium and lactose-free.

THE EVIDENCE FOR SOY AND OSTEOPOROSIS

Despite the cloud of concern that surrounds hormone replacement therapy, taking estrogen does benefit some of the health issues facing women in menopause. One of those health issues is osteoporosis. Estrogen is able to prevent and treat osteoporosis.[31] It slows down both the rapid bone loss that occurs in the first 5 to 8 years of menopause and the long-term loss of bone that happens to women with estrogen levels that are too low.[32]

Because the structure of isoflavones resembles estrogen, there has been a great deal of excitement that soy will also promote bone health.

Natural Soy and Isoflavones

First, look at some of the evidence gotten from studying animals. Many of these studies have been done with rats, because they are good models for studying osteoporosis. Scientists can remove the rats' ovaries to make them menopausal and give them food that is low in calcium. Unless something is done to prevent it, these rats will develop osteoporosis. The scientists can then divide the animals into two groups and feed soy or isoflavones to half of them. The other half does not get any soy or isoflavones. After the study is over, the scientists do a bone density or other tests for measuring bone loss on the two groups of rats, and then compare the results. This is a very good model for studying the effects of a food or a medicine or just about anything on osteoporosis.

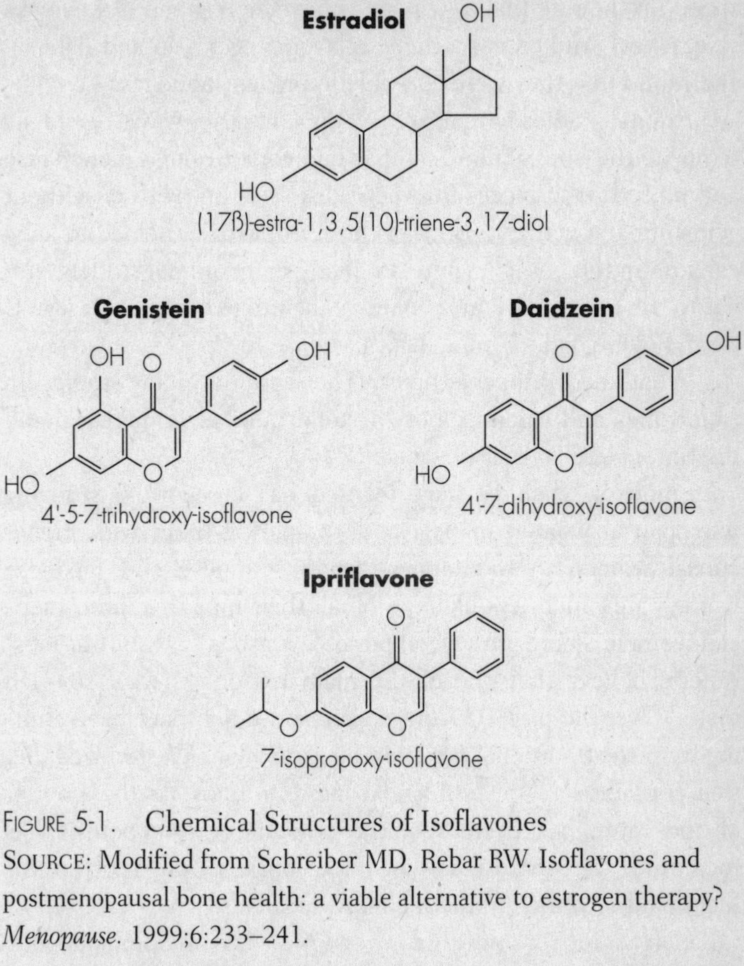

Estradiol

(17ß)-estra-1,3,5(10)-triene-3,17-diol

Genistein

4'-5-7-trihydroxy-isoflavone

Daidzein

4'-7-dihydroxy-isoflavone

Ipriflavone

7-isopropoxy-isoflavone

FIGURE 5-1.   Chemical Structures of Isoflavones
SOURCE: Modified from Schreiber MD, Rebar RW. Isoflavones and postmenopausal bone health: a viable alternative to estrogen therapy? *Menopause*. 1999;6:233–241.

Using this model, scientists proved that a diet containing soy protein prevents bone loss.[33] The same group of scientists did another study and proved that it was the isoflavones within the soy protein that caused the bone protection—when they took the isoflavones out of the soy protein, it no longer prevented bone loss.[34] Other studies showed that just giving genistein by itself could slow down bone loss.[35, 36] Another group found that genistein could not only slow down bone loss but it could also speed up the rate that new bone is formed. A group of Japanese researchers studied two other isoflavones, genistin and daidzin, and found that they were also able to prevent bone loss.[37]

Animal studies have also been done in other ways. Scientists removed the bones from rats that had gone through menopause and placed bone pieces into petri dishes either with or without genistein and genistin. Both of these isoflavones helped to keep calcium in the bone.[38] There are many more animal studies similar to the ones I have mentioned. Taken together the message is clear. Soy is good for bone health.

What about human studies? There are not many studies on isoflavones and calcium, but the total number is increasing all the time. Here is what is available.

Some of what we have learned has come from studying menopausal women in Asia and comparing them with menopausal women in the United States. Chinese and Japanese women are much less likely to break their hips than are American women. There are several possible reasons for this, but most experts believe that one of the main reasons is their soy-rich diet.[39] Over the past 10 years, Japanese women have been shifting from the traditional Japanese diet to a more Westernized diet that contains less soy and isoflavone-rich foods. As the amount of soy eaten has decreased, the amount of osteoporosis has increased. Osteoporosis is now becoming a serious problem for menopausal women in the Japanese society.[40]

Can adding soy to the diet reverse bone loss and promote bone health? One of the best studies that tried to answer this question was done on a group of 66 postmenopausal women (ages 39 to 83 years) who were asked to eat 40 grams of soy protein each day that contained either 55 mg or 90 mg of isoflavones. All the women had a bone-density test done before starting and at the end of 6 months. The results were compared with a group of women who took a placebo.[41] The 90-mg-per-day group faired best, and, just as in the animal studies, isoflavones helped these women protect their bones. In fact, the women actually showed a significant increase in the bone density of their spines and a slight increase in the bone density of their hips and other bones measured.

Another group of scientists did a similar study in 65 women who were perimenopausal (ages 41 to 61 years). These women in the study were given 40 grams of soy protein each day that contained either 80 mg of isoflavones or 4.4 mg of isoflavones.[42] The women had a bone-density test done both before the study began and 24 weeks later. Those who took the 80 mg per day of isoflavones in their soy protein significantly slowed down their rate of bone loss over the time of the study. Those who ate soy protein that contained only small amounts of isoflavones (4.4 mg per day) had much more bone loss, but not as much as the women who did not eat any soy. This study really suggests that soy protein helps prevent bone loss a little bit, but it is the isoflavones that really do the job.

A few other studies on postmenopausal women have also helped to prove soy is beneficial for bone health. In one of those reports, postmenopausal women who each day ate 45 grams of soy-enriched bread increased their bone density compared with women who did not eat the soy.[43] Only one study did not show an effect of soy on bone density.[44] But in another study, 33 women were asked to eat either 60 grams a day of soy protein or a placebo for 3 months and have their urine tested for markers of bone loss.[45] Lower levels in the urine mean less bone loss. The women who took soy had less bone loss! All together these studies support the notion that soy, and in particular the isoflavones, slow bone loss and offer women an alternative to estrogen.

Synthetic Soy—Ipriflavone

Studies on naturally occurring soy have been so promising that several synthetic soy products were developed. The best-known and most studied synthetic isoflavone is ipriflavone—a name that closely resembles isoflavone. It was first manufactured in 1969 and has a chemical structure that is similar to soy isoflavones. Since then it has been used in many patients, primarily in Italy and Japan. It is also available in the United States as a supplement. Like the naturally occurring isoflavones, ipriflavone appears to be useful and safe for treating bone health in menopausal women. Here are some of the studies that make me think that is so.

Once again, most of the studies were done in rats that had their ovaries removed. But this time they were treated either with or without ipriflavone. Very high doses of ipriflavone reduced bone loss just as natural isoflavones did.[46] It worked even better if the animals were started on the ipriflavone 7 days before they had their ovaries removed. Other types of study designs have also been done and all of them show that ipriflavone can slow down bone loss.[47, 48]

There are also quite a few human studies using ipriflavone. Almost all of them have been done in Europe and Japan where the medication has been available for a long time. Most of the first studies were not done too accurately because they did not compare the women who took the medicine with women who did not.[49] Later studies were designed better, so we have more confidence in them.

In a study of 100 women who had fibroids (benign muscle tumors of the uterus), their doctors treated them with 6 months of a medicine that stopped their ovaries from working while they were taking it. That made them temporarily menopausal. Just as in naturally occurring menopause, many women who take this medication for 6 months develop osteoporosis. To stop the osteoporosis from happening, the doctors also gave some of the patients 500 mg of calcium and 600 mg of ipriflavone each day. Some other women did not get the ipriflavone and calcium. None of the women given ipriflavone and calcium developed osteoporosis but the others did.[50]

This same group of doctors also treated 32 women who went through menopause because they had their ovaries removed by surgery.[51] After surgery, half of the women were given 600 mg of ipriflavone and 500 mg of calcium daily, while the other women were given only the calcium. As you might have expected, ipriflavone plus calcium prevented bone loss—something calcium alone could not completely do.

Ipriflavone also prevents bone loss in women just beginning to go through menopause and in women who have already gone through menopause.[52, 53] It also helps to build bone back up in menopausal women who already have lost a significant amount of bone.[54] Adding calcium and vitamin D to the ipriflavone seems to make it even more effective.[55] About 1 in 7 women who take ipriflavone will have some type of reaction to the medication. Negative reactions, 8% of the time, will be gastrointestinal complaints. It is not entirely clear how ipriflavone works to promote bone health, but part of its effectiveness comes from the fact that the body converts it into the natural isoflavone daidzein.[56]

PRESCRIPTION FOR SOY AND BONE HEALTH

The best way to keep your bones strong is to have a healthy lifestyle throughout your life. Exercise, eat a varied diet, and limit animal fat and salt. The best exercise to protect your bones is walking for up to an hour or training with weights for 45 minutes at least 3 times a week. Having said all that, soy can serve as an important alternative in helping to prevent osteoporosis if you do not take estrogen. Soy is also a useful addition to estrogen. The average daily dose for soy protein should be 40 to 80 grams each day; for isoflavones, 50 to 100 mg daily; and for ipriflavone, 200 mg three times daily. Add 500 to 1,200 mg daily of calcium, 400 to 800 mg of vitamin D, and 200 to 600 mg of magnesium daily to strengthen your bones that much more.

chapter 6

SOY AND HEART DISEASE

We have known for a long time that coronary heart disease rates are lower in Japan, where soy consumption is common, than it is in Western countries. The chances of dying of heart disease is sixfold lower for Japanese men and eightfold lower for Japanese women than it is for their American counterparts.[1] Heart disease kills more Americans than any other ailment—more than cancer, accidents, and diabetes combined. The actual numbers exceed 2,600 Americans each day. That's more than 100 people per hour. In 1997, $26.9 billion in payments were made to Medicare beneficiaries for hospital expenses due to cardiovascular (high blood pressure, coronary heart disease including heart disease and chest pain, stroke and congestive heart failure) problems— an average of $7,873 per discharge.[2] The 1998 estimated total direct and indirect costs of cardiovascular disease in the United States were over $298 billion.[3] Estimates state that 2 in 1,000 Americans will suffer a heart attack each year and one third of them will die.

Although heart disease is typically considered a man's disease, that really is not the case. More than 1 in 5 women have some form of cardiovascular disease. By the time she is 65 that likelihood increases to 1 in 3.[4] African-American women are at even greater risk than these averages.

Women tend to develop heart disease about 10 years later than men when they are over the age of 65, but approximately

20,000 women who are younger—a third of them under 55—die of heart attacks each year.[5] As women reach menopause, the rates of heart attack for men and women narrow. By age 75, the rate of heart attacks in women actually surpasses the rates in men. Most alarming are surveys showing less than 10% of women realize cardiovascular disease is the number one killer of women.

If nothing could be done to change these large numbers, all this discussion would not matter. But heart disease can in part be prevented through lifestyle changes. Estimates are that if all major cardiovascular disease were eliminated, life expectancy would rise by almost 7 years. Compare this to, if all forms of cancer were eliminated, the life span gain would be 3 years. Concerning diet and heart disease, there is more involved than simply avoiding fat and eating fiber. Soy can play an important role in lowering blood cholesterol and the risk of developing heart disease.

UNDERSTANDING HEART DISEASE

The heart is a pump made of special muscle called myocardium. It is a little larger than your fist and its four chambers are divided vertically into two sides by a wall. The right side pumps blood to your lungs to receive oxygen and to rid itself of carbon dioxide. The refreshed blood returns to the left side of the heart and is immediately pumped out into your arteries, sending oxygen and nutrients throughout your body and returning carbon dioxide to the heart and lungs to exchange for a fresh supply of oxygen. Since the heart is a muscle, it needs oxygen, too, which it gets as blood passes through the coronary arteries. Each time the heart beats we feel it as a pulse. On average, the heart beats about 100,000 times each day, pumping about 2,000 gallons of blood in the process.

At birth, our arteries are clean and very elastic. With each heartbeat the arteries expand and contract back down to their original size, sending a small wave of blood farther along its journey. Clean, elastic arteries make the heart's job much easier. Beginning with childhood,[6] plaque deposits begin to attach to our arteries, making their walls less elastic and making the heart pump much harder to get the same job done. As the arteries narrow and their walls harden, blood pressure increases, just as water pressure in a hose increases when the end is blocked.

The high blood pressure (hypertension) that results is a risk factor for heart disease. Hypertension affects 20.3% of American women aged 20 to 74.[7] Here is how the most recent percentages break down by age:[8]

TABLE 6-1. HIGH BLOOD PRESSURE IN WOMEN

Age	Percentage Affected
20–34	3.4
35–44	12.7
45–54	25.1
55–64	44.2
65–74	60.8
>75	77.3

SOURCE: Health United States 2000, Centers for Disease Control and Prevention, National Center for Health Statistics.

Hardening of the arteries is called atherosclerosis. During the Korean War, nearly 75% of 2,000 American soldiers killed in battle, whose average age was 22, already had significant atherosclerosis.[9] Cholesterol is a major contributor to this problem, but other substances and lifestyle activities can also contribute.

If atherosclerosis leads to complete blockage of an artery, no blood can flow through it, and the part of the body depending on that artery for oxygen and nutrition can die. If this happens to an artery in the heart—a condition called coronary heart disease—a portion of the heart will die and the person will have a myocardial infarction, or heart attack. Studies performed by Dr. Dean Ornish have shown that strict diets low in fat combined with exercise can actually reverse atherosclerosis.[10] There are, in fact, several risk factors that you can change to lower your risk of heart disease.

MODIFIABLE RISK FACTORS FOR HEART DISEASE
Smoking

According to the American Heart Association, smoking may account for one fifth of cardiovascular deaths and is the leading preventable cause of heart disease in women.[11] Smoking as few as one to four cigarettes daily doubles a woman's risk of cardiovascular heart disease and smoking twenty or more cigarettes doubles to quadruples it. More than half of all heart attacks in middle-aged women are related to cigarette smoking. Cigarettes thicken the blood, which can lead to clots, and raise carbon monoxide levels in the blood, which robs the heart and other tissues of oxygen, and the nicotine narrows the coronary arteries, which raises blood pressure causing the heart to work harder. The good news is that if you stop smoking, your risk of a heart attack goes down immediately, reaching the level of a nonsmoker by 5 to 10 years.

Obesity and Fat Distribution

Overweight women, especially those who carry their weight on their abdomen and upper body (the so-called apple shape) are at greater risk of developing heart disease than slim women or those whose weight is primarily on their hips and thighs (the so-called pear shape). From the viewpoint of heart disease, the hip-to-waist ratio for women approaching menopause should be less than 0.8.

Obesity also increases the risk of high blood pressure and diabetes—two additional independent risk factors for heart disease. I discussed body mass index (BMI) in Chapter 1. This number is calculated by dividing your weight in kilograms by the square of your height in meters. A desirable BMI is less than 25. Women with a BMI over 29 have three times the risk of cardiovascular heart disease of lean women with a BMI under 21.[12] The same study showed that women who are moderately overweight (BMI of 25 to 28.9) have almost double the risk of heart disease. Even women who are not overweight but who gained weight during adulthood (most do) or whose weight is near the top of the normal range will have a slight increased risk of heart disease.[13] Recent surveys show that more than half of Americans are overweight (65.5% of men and 52.7% of women ages 45 to 54). It is much better to try and keep our weight stable. Frequent weight fluctuations from yo-yo dieting are also a risk factor for heart disease.[14] Eating a healthful diet in moderation can go a long way to lowering your risk of heart disease.

Sedentary Lifestyle

The American Heart Association considers a sedentary lifestyle to be an independent risk factor for heart disease. It is something that doesn't get enough attention in this age of computers and television, but not getting enough exercise increases your risk of developing heart disease from 1.5 to 2.4 times—about the same amount as increased cholesterol levels, hypertension, or cigarette smoking. Only about 1 in 5 Americans report engaging in regular, sustained exercise of any intensity for 30 minutes or more 5 days a week. Unfortunately, fewer women than men exercise regularly.

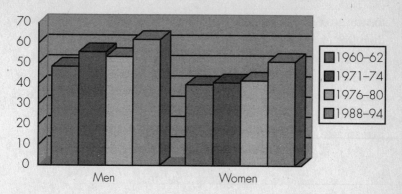

FIGURE 6-1.   Age-Adjusted (2000 Standard) Prevalence of
Overweight in Americans Ages 20 to 74 by Sex and Survey
NOTE: Overweight is defined as a BMI of 25 and higher.
SOURCE: Respective health examination surveys, Centers for Disease
Control, National Center for Health Statistics.

Stress

All of us know how bad stress can make us feel. If it accumu-
lates over time, all parts of the body are affected—the brain, the
heart, the blood vessels, and the muscles. The effects can be so
great that one study suggested stress is responsible for an
increased likelihood of death in a spouse whose partner has died
within the previous 6 months. Suicide, accidents, or alcohol-
related events were likely causes of death in these cases, and
men were more at risk than women.

Mental stress is just as likely to cause angina as physical
stress and may even pose a higher risk for heart attacks. One
example of this was the significantly increased number of heart
attacks that took place during the 1996 Los Angeles earthquake.
Only a few deaths were related to physical exertion. Stress
causes the heart to beat harder and faster and causes the blood
vessels to narrow. You can see how this is a perfect setup for
reducing the amount of blood to the heart and possibly causing a

heart attack. Stress also sets the stage for abnormal heart rhythms and makes the blood become stickier (possibly in preparation for a potential injury), which in turn increases the risk of developing a blood clot. The sudden increases in blood pressure caused by stress may, over time, damage the inner lining of blood vessels and contribute to atherosclerosis. Soy cannot eliminate stress, but it may be able to help your body absorb it.

Diabetes Mellitus

Diabetes has become an epidemic in this country. Another person is diagnosed with the disease every 40 seconds. According to the Centers for Disease Control (CDC), that is a 33% increase in the number of people diagnosed between 1990 and 1998. The rise crossed all races and age groups, but was sharpest, about 70%, among people ages 30 to 39. The American Diabetes Association uses the criteria of a fasting blood glucose level of 126 milligrams per deciliter (mg/dL) or higher to define diabetes, and women entering or in menopause are at a high risk of developing diabetes.[15] Fast foods, especially those high in fat, combined with an increased consumption of sugar and a sedentary lifestyle, have taken their toll. More than 16 million Americans suffer from diabetes. The risk for Mexican Americans and non-Hispanic blacks is almost twice that for whites.[16]

Diabetes is more common in women than in men, and its effects on the risk of developing cardiovascular disease are greater. Diabetes increases the chances of developing cardiovascular heart disease by threefold in men. In women, having diabetes may increase their risk from fourfold to as much as sevenfold.[17] The risk that a person with diabetes who has never had a heart attack is the same as the risk for a nondiabetic person who already has had a heart attack having a second. Diabetes can also damage the retina of the eyes, making it the leading cause of blindness in working-age adults in the United States. It causes kidney damage and damages the nerves of the body, leading to an increased risk of leg amputation. Soy is an excellent food choice for people suffering from diabetes because it can help to reduce some of the damaging effects of this chronic disease.

Cholesterol

Everyone has heard of cholesterol, a fatlike substance that circulates in the blood. Cholesterol is also called lipids. Because fats do not mix well in blood, which is mostly water, cholesterol must be carried throughout the bloodstream by protein molecules called lipoproteins or proteins that carry lipids. The three major types of lipoproteins are:

- Low-density lipoprotein (LDL), which carries 60% to 70% of cholesterol in the blood and takes it to your body's tissues. LDL is called bad cholesterol because it contributes to the formation of plaque in the blood vessels.
- High-density lipoprotein (HDL), which carries 20% to 30% of total cholesterol. HDL is called good cholesterol because it helps to remove excess cholesterol by bringing it back to the liver where it is broken down and eliminated from the body.
- Very-low-density lipoprotein (VLDL), which carries the remaining 10% to 15% of cholesterol and most of the triglycerides.

The Framingham study, which began in Framingham, Massachusetts, in 1949 with 5,000 men and women and which still continues today, taught us the significance of cholesterol for heart disease. Fifty-year-old men who have blood cholesterol levels higher than 295 mg/dL are 9 times more likely to have a heart attack as those with cholesterol levels of 200 mg/dL. The point was driven home even further by the fact that no one in the study with a cholesterol level below 150 mg/dL ever had a heart attack.

More than 50 million American women have lipid levels in the undesirable range: 51% have total cholesterol levels above 200 mg/dL and roughly half of those (20%) have total cholesterol levels that exceed 240 mg/dL.[18] Unfortunately, nearly two thirds of post-menopausal women who need treatment to lower their cholesterol are not receiving any.[19] Which is really too bad, because for every 1 mg/dL reduction in LDL there is a 2% relative risk reduction, and for every 1 mg/dL increase in HDL there is a 3% to 5% reduction.[20] Fortunately, a healthy lifestyle combined with a low-fat diet and soy can help to lower cholesterol—so much so that in 1999 the Food and Drug Administration approved this as a claim.

CHOLESTEROL AND DIET

There is so much talk about cholesterol that one is left with the opinion that even a little is bad. However, cholesterol is essential for life. Every cell in the body needs it, and it plays an

TABLE 6-2. LIPID LEVELS AND RISK OF HEART DISEASE

	Total Cholesterol (mg/dL)	HDL (mg/dL)	LDL (mg/dL)	Triglycerides (mg/dL)
Desirable	<200	35	<130	<200
Undesirable	≥200	<35	≥130	≥200
Borderline high risk	200–239	—	130–159	200–400
High risk	>240	—	≥160	400–1,000
Very high risk	—	—	—	>1,000

NOTE: HDL ≥60 mg/dL is a negative risk. Optimal HDL may be ≥45 mg/dL in women.

important role in making the hormones estrogen, progesterone, and testosterone. We also use cholesterol as part of the membrane surrounding our body's nerve cells and for making vitamin D when our skin is exposed to sunlight. Although linoleic acid (an omega-6 fatty acid) and alpha-linolenic acid (an omega-3 fatty acid) are essential fats, that is, we cannot make them and must eat them, our liver and intestines are quite capable of making cholesterol. Our bodies try to keep everything in balance, so that if we eat more cholesterol, we make less and vice versa. However, if our diets contain too much cholesterol, eventually the system breaks down and cholesterol begins to accumulate in our bloodstream. We now know that for every 100 milligrams (mg) of cholesterol we eat per 1,000 calories in our diet, our LDL cholesterol rises by about 8 points. Soy, and a more vegetarian diet in general, can play an important role in this balance, because cholesterol is only present in animal foods. There is no cholesterol in plants. Every animal cell contains cholesterol. Even lean meat and skinless chicken still contain cholesterol.

SATURATED AND UNSATURATED FAT

Not all fats are the same. There are three types of fat: saturated, monounsaturated, and polyunsaturated. These are all from the fat family called fatty acids. Cholesterol is from another lipid family called sterols. All fats do share something in common; they are made from carbon and hydrogen with a few molecules of oxygen. They differ from each other by the number of carbon atoms and how the atoms are arranged. In a saturated fatty acid all the carbon atoms in the chain are linked to hydrogen atoms at all possible positions. In other words, all the possible positions are saturated with hydrogen. The term unsaturated refers to two carbon atoms with one less hydrogen atom between them, so that there is a double bond between the two carbons. Monounsaturated means that there is one double bond. Polyunsaturated means that there is more than one double bond.

FIGURE 6-2. SATURATED AND UNSATURATED FATS

Saturated Fatty Acid

C-C-C-C-C-C-C-C-C-C-C-C-C-C-C-C-C-C-C

Monounsaturated Fatty Acid

C-C-C-C-C-C-C-C-C=C-C-C-C-C-C-C-C-C-C

Polyunsaturated Fatty Acid

C-C-C-C-C=C-C-C-C=C-C-C-C-C-C-C-C-C

NOTE: Saturated fatty acids have only single (–) bonds between carbon atoms (C). Monounsaturated fatty acids contain a single double (=) bond between two carbon atoms. Polyunsaturated fatty acids have more than one double bond. Although double bonds cause the molecule to bend, these are all shown straight for simplicity.
SOURCE: Modified from Schmidt MA. *Smart Fats*. Berkeley, Calif.: Frog Ltd; 1997.

Saturated fats are usually solid at room temperature. Unsaturated fats are typically liquid at room temperature. Foods high in saturated fat include meat, dairy products, and eggs. Coconut and palm-kernel oil as well as chocolate also contain saturated fat. Saturated fats raise cholesterol levels even more than eating cholesterol. Saturated fats are a potential problem because they block liver receptors that remove LDL cholesterol from the bloodstream and contribute to those levels rising.[21] Throughout the world, the more saturated fat that people eat, the higher the rate of heart disease. Keeping your intake of saturated fat to a minimum will go a long way to lowering your risk of heart disease. Given this information, it is amazing that many fast food franchises have found their way into the cafeterias of our leading hospitals.

TRANS FATTY ACIDS—ANOTHER WORRISOME FAT

Trans fatty acids were developed to offer an alternative to cholesterol. It was an experiment that did not work out as planned. Trans fatty acids actually increase blood cholesterol. Their impact is somewhere between those of saturated and unsaturated fatty acids. They were actually developed because unsaturated fatty acids are generally a liquid and cannot be used easily to make margarine, shortening, or other solid fats. So a new technique was developed to add hydrogen to vegetable oil. Any food that contains partially hydrogenated fat contains trans fatty acids—and that is the majority of deep fried foods and many packaged and prepared foods such as potato chips, doughnuts, and cookies. Nearly half the fat in a bag of potato chips may occur as trans fatty acids—up to 4.6 grams or nearly 1 teaspoon.[22]

Harvard researchers have found that women consuming high levels of trans fatty acids have 50% greater risk of heart disease than those consuming the least.[23] Some investigators believe that trans fatty acids may even be worse for us than saturated fats.

Neither trans fatty acids nor saturated fat is desirable as the sole source of dietary fat. The goal is to limit their intake to a minimum.

DIETARY THERAPY FOR HEART DISEASE

Although people who have a genetic tendency to high cholesterol levels may need to take a medication to lower their levels and reduce their risk of heart disease, most people with elevated

cholesterol can improve their levels and their risk of heart disease by combining exercise with a healthful diet. Doctors can
encourage their patients to adopt a healthy diet, but according to
a study by the Centers for Disease Control, only 42% of patients
receive advice from their physician to eat low-fat and low-cholesterol foods and increase their physical activity. The good news is
that two thirds of those patients acted on the dietary advice and
61% increased their physical activity.[24]

Incorporating soy in your diet can help you reach normal
LDL levels. The traditional Asian diet contains a steady intake
of soy, primarily in the form of soybean curd (tofu) (47%), fermented soybeans (30%), and soybean paste (11%).[25] The
Asian diet tends to be very low in fat, high in complex carbohydrates, very low in sweets, rich in vegetables and fruits, and
very low in animal products. Low to moderate alcohol consumption is also typical. This translates into about 14% fat,
71% carbohydrates, and 10% protein, with animal protein
accounting for less than 1%. In China, dietary fat intake
increased from 15.9% in 1982 to 21.1% in 1990. Along with
this increase, the incidence of heart disease also increased.[26]
Even this degree of fat is very different from the typical American diet that contains 36% fat, 42% carbohydrates, and 15%
protein, 10% of which is from animals. The importance of a
low-fat diet was most clearly established by Dr. Dean Ornish.
He showed that people whose blood vessels were so severely
blocked that they were recommended for bypass surgery on
their coronary arteries to prevent a heart attack could actually
reverse the blockage and clean their arteries by eating a very-
low-fat (10%), high-carbohydrate diet along with meditation
and exercise. Those who did not change their diets found no
change in their arteries or their arteries kept getting progres-
sively blocked.[27] One of the best ways to get a heart-healthy
diet is by incorporating soy.

BRING ON THE SOY

We have known since the turn of the century that the more animal protein we eat, the greater the risk of atherosclerosis. From many clinical studies we know that lowering the amount of saturated fats reduces the risk of heart disease. These two important points have kept the focus on eating less animal fat instead of shifting the focus to eating *more* vegetable protein, such as soy.

There is now nearly 40 years of medical research showing the benefits of soy protein on lowering cholesterol. Some of the first human studies to make this observation were conducted by researchers trying to prove that soy protein was a good nutritional substitute for meat.[28] In addition to proving that soy protein is an excellent protein alternative to meat, they found that cholesterol levels went down in subjects who ate soy. Nearly a decade later, a study on the effects of soy on cholesterol was done in a group of people who had genetically elevated cholesterol. It was found that soy protein lowered cholesterol levels by 14% in 2 weeks and by 21% in 3 weeks.[29]

Since that time, there have been many studies showing the ability of soy protein to lower cholesterol in people whose cholesterol levels are elevated. A famous one was published in 1995.[30] In that analysis of 38 controlled clinical trials of soy protein, an average consumption of 47 grams of soy protein daily was able to lower serum cholesterol levels an average of 9.3% in 34 of the 38 studies. Overall, if a person has a slightly increased cholesterol level and adds soy to their diet, there is a very good chance that they will find their cholesterol in the normal range after a few months.

What about people whose cholesterol level is normal? Not all studies show that people with a normal cholesterol level can expect soy use to bring their levels even lower. However, at least one study done in premenopausal women found that after 1 month of taking 60 grams of soy protein, cholesterol levels dropped 9.6%, which is almost the same drop as in individuals with elevated cholesterol.[31] Another study found that people with normal cholesterol could expect a significant reduction in their LDL-cholesterol levels from eating soy if they were also eating a high-cholesterol diet. However, eating soy with a low-cholesterol diet did not seem to make a difference.[32] Taken together, these studies tell us that if we have a normal cholesterol level but our diet leaves something to be desired, adding soy offers the best chance of keeping cholesterol normal. Postmenopausal women with normal or mildly elevated cholesterol levels can also benefit from soy protein and expect a similar improvement in their cholesterol levels.[33]

Another recent study in postmenopausal women with elevated cholesterol levels found that soy protein that had the isoflavones removed were not nearly as effective in lowering cholesterol as soy protein with the isoflavones left intact.[34] Although isoflavones are very important in the cholesterol-lowering ability of soy—and I am a strong believer in isoflavone capsules for hot flashes, bone health, and keeping our arteries more elastic—isoflavone capsules alone do not seem to be very effective in lowering cholesterol.[35] But when adjusting your diet is the first line of therapy, eating soy foods is a terrific way to get your cholesterol level down.

How Does Soy Lower Cholesterol?

Although it is clear that soy helps to lower cholesterol, we do not know exactly how this occurs. More than one mechanism may be going on at the same time. For instance, soy increases the rate that cholesterol is cleared from the bloodstream.[36] Getting it out of the body quickly keeps levels lower than they otherwise would be. But other researchers have shown that soy can both slow down the speed at which the body is able to manufacture cholesterol and reduce the amount of cholesterol a person absorbs from their intestinal tract after eating cholesterol.[37] At least some of this is due to the fiber found in soy. About 30% of soy's fiber is soluble. It is called soluble fiber because it is soluble in water. Soluble fiber is present in oat bran, rice bran, fruits, many vegetables, and our good friend soy. Our upper or small intestinal tract cannot digest fiber, so we cannot absorb it there. Instead, the fiber makes its way through our intestinal tract to our colon, where the bacteria there digest it through a process called fermentation. The process of fermentation produces a number of substances that help to lower cholesterol.[38] Soy fiber is most effective in lowering cholesterol in people whose cholesterol levels are elevated.

In their excellent book *The Simple Soybean and Your Health,* Doctors Messina and Setchell offer another explanation—that the amino acids in soy are able to change the levels of the hormone insulin and thyroid hormone, which in turn lowers cholesterol levels.[39] It may work like this: Soybeans and other plant foods are high in the amino acids glycine and arginine, both of which lower insulin levels in the blood. Because insulin stimulates the liver to make cholesterol, lower levels of insulin help to keep cholesterol levels down.[40] Animal proteins are just the opposite—low in arginine and glycine. They also happen to be high in lysine, an amino acid that raises insulin levels. These facts help to explain why even eating a lean-meat diet cannot lower cholesterol levels as much as eating a more vegetarian diet. In fact, diets that use plant foods as the predominant food source are about twice as effective at lowering cholesterol as diets that include lean meat. Doctors Messina and Setchell point out an interesting irony of this information. Many nutritionists are often critical of plant protein diets for the very reason that they are low in lysine—a fact that may really be a benefit. All of this makes soy add up to a great dietary way of helping to keep cholesterol levels in check.

Other Ways Soy Benefits Your Heart

Lowering cholesterol is not the only major benefit of soy. Soy may also help lower blood pressure. In one animal model, mice with high blood pressure were fed a diet high in salt to make their blood pressure even higher. When soy was added to the diet, their blood pressure values lowered.[41] Although soy did not lower high-normal blood pressure values in one human study,[42] another human study did show that a soy dietary supplement, which was given twice daily to 51 perimenopausal women with normal blood pressures, was able to significantly decrease diastolic blood pressure.[43] It will take some more studies before we have the final answer on soy and blood pressure.

A team of researchers led by Dr. Tom Clarkson at Wake Forest University has done a lot of work in cynomolgus (a particular type of monkey) monkeys to understand how soy might benefit humans. One area of investigation has been on soy's effect on coronary arteries—the blood vessels of the heart. Their studies and those of others point to soy as playing an important role in keeping our heart blood vessel walls free of plaque and in helping them to remain elastic. In monkeys that have had their ovaries removed to make them menopausal, it was found that significantly less plaque formed in their coronary arteries if they were fed soy containing its isoflavones than if they were fed soy with isoflavones removed.[44] They also found that blood vessels remained more elastic in monkeys fed soy—just as elastic as those given estrogen and even more elastic than those given estrogen plus medroxyprogesterone acetate.[45]

Studies in humans also show that soy can make blood vessels more elastic.[46] Soy isoflavones (80 mg per day for 5 to 10 weeks) given to 21 women aged 46 to 67 made their arteries 26% more elastic compared with placebo.[47] These results are nearly identical with the results in postmenopausal women treated with long-term hormone replacement therapy[48] and reinforce similar results in primate studies.[49]

At least some of this beneficial effect of soy is due to the isoflavone genistein that has been found to slow down new blood vessel growth (antiangiogenesis) and slow down blood clot formation.[50] Add to this the fact that relatively low doses of isoflavones are also strong antioxidants that protect LDL-C from oxidation and you have a terrific food to help you maintain a healthy heart.[51] Since soy does not have a negative effect on the uterine lining and it results in blood vessels being more elastic than does progesterone, I and others believe that taking estrogen together with soy might be preferable to taking estrogen plus progesterone for women who want to take estrogen and who have not had a hysterectomy.[52]

How Much Soy Do You Need?

If eating soy does not appeal to you, but you want to get soy into your body for its healthy heart benefits, do you have to throw away your knife and fork and never look at a serving of animal protein again? The answer is no. Even a small amount of soy in your diet can help. In fact, the Food and Drug Administration in October 1999 approved the health claim that a dietary intake of at least 25 grams per day of soy protein is capable of lowering cholesterol, if taken in conjunction with a healthy lifestyle and a diet low in saturated fat. How much is 25 grams? Considering a pound is 454 grams or 16 ounces, it's about $\frac{1}{18}$ of a pound, less than 1 ounce. The North American Menopause Society further suggests that if your goals are to make your arteries more elastic, 40 to 80 mg per day of isoflavones should do the trick; for antioxidant effects on lipids, 10 mg per day.

Consider the following study done on patients who were asked to follow the American Heart Association's diet for 4 weeks and afterward had only minor reductions in their cholesterol levels.[53] When they added soy to their diets but kept everything else the same, their LDL-cholesterol levels dropped by 33% after 4 weeks and even more after 4 months.

If you really want to improve your heart health, do not smoke, try to control your weight, exercise, and watch your blood pressure. Also, replace as much of your daily animal protein intake as you can with soy.

chapter 7

SOY AND CANCER

Cancer is probably the most frightening word in the English language. One in every 3 Americans will have cancer at some point in their lives, and it will claim the life of nearly 1 in every 4 Americans (22%). Only heart disease kills more people in the United States. The average person who develops cancer will lose almost 15 years from his or her life. Recent statistics show that in the United States there are more than 1.5 million new cancer cases each year and more than 550,000 deaths occur each year due to cancer. Unfortunately, the number of cancer deaths increases steadily. According to the American Institute for Cancer Research (AICR), more than 10 million new cancer cases occur around the world each year.

In a landmark report from the AICR in 1997, a panel of leading scientists analyzed over 4,500 research studies from around the world and concluded that what we eat (or do not eat) could reduce cancer rates significantly. If people were to change their dietary habits to include 5 or more servings of fruits and vegetables each day, cancer rates could decline by as much as 20%. For certain cancers, a change of diet could even have a greater effect. They estimated that as many as half of all breast cancers, 1 in every 3 cases of lung cancer, and 3 in every 4 cases of colon and rectal cancer could be prevented with more healthful diets.[1] Believe it or not, less than one fourth of United States citizens actually eat 5 servings of fruits and vegetables each day, even if we count ketchup as one of the servings.

TABLE 7-1. ESTIMATED NEW CANCER CASES AND DEATHS—2002 ESTIMATES

New Cancer Cases by Site and Sex		Cancer Deaths by Site and Sex	
Male	Female	Male	Female
Prostate 189,000	Breast 203,500	Lung & bronchus 89,200	Lung & bronchus 65,700
Lung & bronchus 90,200	Lung & bronchus 79,200	Prostate 30,200	Breast 39,600
Colon & rectum 72,600	Colon & rectum 75,700	Colon & rectum 27,800	Colon & rectum 28,800
Urinary bladder 41,500	Uterine corpus 39,300	Pancreas 14,500	Pancreas 15,200
Non-Hodgkin's lymphoma 28,200	Non-Hodgkin's lymphoma 25,700	Non-Hodgkin's lymphoma 12,700	Ovary 13,900
All sites 637,500	All sites 647,400	All sites 288,200	All sites 267,300

SOURCE: Cancer Statistics, 2002. *CA Cancer J Clin* 2002;52:23–47. Excludes basal and squamous cell skin cancer and in situ carcinomas except urinary bladder.

There is even more good news if you include soy in your diet. Soy foods are a rich source of anticarcinogens—substances that are able to prevent or control cancer. As you read on in this chapter, you will find that soy is one of the best dietary choices you can make for avoiding cancer.

WHAT IS CANCER?

Part of what makes cancer frightening is the fact that some of a person's own cells have turned potentially lethal. What is it that makes cells that normally divide in a very controlled way suddenly get out of control?

Cells are the basic units of all living things. The human body contains some 100 trillion individual cells and these make up the tissues and organs of our bodies. As Dr. Geoffrey Cooper of

FIGURE 7-1. AGE-ADJUSTED CANCER DEATH RATES, FEMALES BY SITE, U.S., 1930–1996

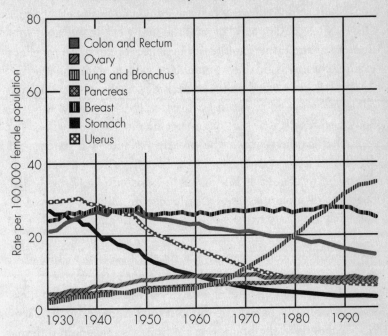

NOTE: Per 100,000, age-adjusted to the 1970 U.S. standard population. Uterine cancer death rates are for uterine cervix and uterine corpus combined.

SOURCE: U.S. Mortality Public Use Data Tapes 1960–1996, U.S. Mortality Volumes 1930–1959, National Center for Health Statistics, Centers for Disease Control and Prevention, 1999. American Cancer Society, Surveillance Research.

Harvard Medical School explains it, each of these cells is programmed to perform a specialized task that is important to the person as a whole, much as each individual performs specialized tasks that contribute to the common good of society.[2] Like the individual humans who make up society, who grow and reproduce, individual cells are also able to grow and reproduce. Each cell's growth and reproduction is carefully controlled, so that one parent cell divides into two daughter cells. Some cells such as nerve cells seldom divide when the individual becomes an adult. Others such as skin and hair and the lining of the intestine continue to divide rather rapidly throughout a lifetime. An excellent example of this is the blood-producing cells of the bone marrow. About 1 trillion blood cells die each day in the average normal adult and must be replaced by division. In a controlled way, the body restores itself as part of an ongoing process.

What happens when the orderly fashion of a parent cell dividing to make two daughter cells goes haywire? The answer is the origin of cancer. It is a process of uncontrolled growth that begins to divide under its own influence, forming new abnormal cells that grow into masses of tissue called tumors.

Not all tumors are cancer. A tumor can be benign and relatively harmless, unable to invade nearby tissue or to spread to distant sites. An example of a benign tumor is the common skin wart. Benign tumors are almost never life threatening unless they occur in places that are difficult to operate on, such as specific locations in the brain. But if a tumor is malignant it develops the ability to invade nearby tissue and eventually to spread to other parts of the body, either through the lymph glands or through the bloodstream. Over time the cancer cells divide more rapidly than the normal cells of a particular organ. The cancer cells crowd out normal cells so the organ can no longer work properly.

The fact that cancer is believed to originate from one cell that becomes abnormal is frightening, considering there are about 100 trillion cells in the body, and each one of them divides approximately 10,000 trillion times over a person's lifetime.[3] Fortunately, when a cell first begins to divide abnormally, it is not yet cancer. It must go through a series of steps and changes that eventually end in the formation of cancer.

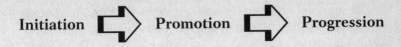

FIGURE 7-2.

Cancer—A Genetic Accident

With all the talk about the genome project, you probably have heard about DNA, the molecular bits of protein material that make up our genetic destiny and carry a code that determines what we will inherit and how our cells will function. DNA is made of a double helix, two molecular-size strands of DNA that are paired together and twisted in a spiral. Each parent cell that divides passes along its DNA to each of its daughter cells. It is the process that allows the cells in each organ of the body to act like the parent organ and not some other type of tissue. Breast cells make breasts, ovary cells make ovaries, colon cells make colons, and so on. The cells in each organ are programmed with a specific destiny that allows them to act in a precise way. This planned distinction of one cell from another is called differentiation. Each type of cell is different from another. Cancer cells lose their ability to follow their programmed destiny, which is to carry out a specific function, to reproduce, and then to die. They become more and more undifferentiated and primitive in their appearance and behavior. They continue to divide but they do not die, becoming almost immortal. The more undifferentiated the cells become, the more lethal the cancer. Given the fact that every hour of the day 600 million of our cells are dividing, an occasional accident should not be a surprise. Depending on the type of mistake, a cell could turn into cancer.[4]

Some of our genes are intended to stimulate a cell to grow and divide, while other genes inhibit cell division. These genes have a significant potential effect on causing cancer. Two in particular are proto-oncogenes and oncogenes.[5] Proto-oncogenes are normal genes that help to regulate cell growth and differentiation. Like all normal processes in the body, they work in a very programmed way and know when to start and when to stop affecting a particular cell. The problems begin when a particular proto-oncogene becomes mutated, meaning damaged. It suddenly stops working as a helpful regulator of normal cell function and instead becomes an oncogene—a cancer-causing gene. There are now approximately 100 oncogenes and roughly half of them produce a protein called tyrosine kinase that acts as an enzyme to speed up cell communication and alter its activity. Soy contains tyrosine kinase inhibitors and that may explain one way in which soy helps to prevent cancer.[6] In fact, genistein is a specific inhibitor of protein tyrosine kinase.[7]

Carcinogenesis—The Evolution of a Cancer Cell

Cancer is not a single mistake, but a series of errors that happen to a cell. Depending on the type of cancer, these stages may happen over a short period of time or over a long period of time. Much is still being learned, but here is a brief review of carcinogenesis.

STAGE I—INITIATION

Most genes are not involved in the regulation of a cell's growth and division. Mistakes in those genes typically do not cause any serious harm. But when proto-oncogenes are altered by a mutation and turn into oncogenes, that cell has taken the first step toward becoming a cancer cell. There are still at least two more steps to go through, but this first change is called initiation. Substances that cause mutations that lead to cancer are called carcinogens. Some viruses, high-dose radiation, tobacco, and a wide range of chemicals including benzidine, aflatoxin, radon, and naphthylamine are examples of carcinogens. They all have one thing in common—

they react with a cell's DNA to cause a mutation that alters the function of genes critical to regulating a cell's growth.

In addition to the carcinogens listed above, some components that are in food may also be carcinogens. These include nitrates, which are high in foods such as hot dogs; some food preservatives and colorings; and the carbon found on the skin of meats cooked on an open flame. Even some foods found in nature, such as horseradish and black pepper, may contain carcinogens. Fortunately, our cells are not completely defenseless. They contain checking mechanisms that are able to correct these errors if they find them before the cell divides. Once an initiated cell divides, the mistake is permanent.

With so many possible exposures and so many cells dividing, it is almost impossible to avoid or catch them all. Most of us may have some cells in our bodies that have undergone initiation. The good news is that for cancer to occur, the initiated cell must be promoted, which is the second stage of carcinogenesis.

STAGE II—PROMOTION

Initiation is a permanent step. Once a cell is initiated it cannot reverse the damage that has occurred to its DNA. Each initiated parent cell in turn divides and passes on this initiation to its two daughter cells. But these cells must come in contact with other chemicals that increase its rate of cell division—a process called proliferation. Substances that do this are called promoting agents, which is why this stage is called promotion. Promoting agents are not carcinogens because they do not cause initiation. But they do make initiated cells divide at a faster rate. Unless a promoting agent stimulates an initiated cell, it will not go on toward cancer. A portion of the initiated cells may begin dividing so fast that some of them start to look different from the parent cell—more undifferentiated. The more abnormal a cell looks, the more likely it is to turn into cancer. Some examples of promoting agents are the hormone estrogen and dietary fat. There is one very important difference between initiation and promotion. Promotion is reversible. In most cases, a promoter must be used repeatedly before the final changes occur that lead to cancer. That is why changing a lifetime of poor eating habits and switching to a more healthful diet can stop the proliferation of initiated cells, even if the process is well along the way.[8] Soy isoflavones have the ability to slow down this cell proliferation.[9]

STAGE III—PROGRESSION

At some point there is no turning back and cells that have been initiated and promoted turn into cancer. This is called progression. Cancer cells are able to spread locally and invade nearby tissues. They can metastasize or spread to distant parts of the body. As cancer cells invade and grow, they need blood nutrients and oxygen just as normal tissues do. To accomplish this, the cancer will develop its own network of blood vessels, a process known as angiogenesis. Soy goes once more to the rescue because it contains substances that can stop angiogenesis.[10]

SOY—A SOURCE OF ANTICARCINOGENS

Just as there are carcinogens that encourage the development of cancer, there are also anticarcinogens—substances that discourage the development of cancer. People in countries where soy is a major component of diet, primarily in Asia, have tremendously lower rates of breast cancer than do people in the United States. Colon and rectal cancer rates are also lower among people who eat soy. The reasons for this are many. Certainly, people in Asian countries eat less animal protein, less fat, and more fiber. But even when these factors are taken into consideration, eating soy foods has been found to be protective against cancer. That is because soy foods are a rich source of anticarcinogens. In fact, soybeans contain a number of anticarcinogens that are present in large enough amounts that eating soy can be beneficial to your health.

Protease Inhibitors

Proteases are enzymes that digest other proteins. Cancer cells use proteases to digest the walls of tissues and blood vessels as they attack normal tissue en route to metastasizing. In fact, the higher the level of proteases a particular cancer cell secretes, the more likely it is to spread. From this brief explanation you can see how important it is to identify ways of slowing down or stopping protease. Anticarcinogenic protease inhibitors do not affect normal cell division or any other normal cell function.[11] This makes soy's protease inhibitors nontoxic. In addition, protease inhibitors offer some protection from radiation and free radicals.

One specific soybean-derived protease inhibitor is called Bowman-Birk inhibitor (BBI). It seems to have such promise in combating cancer that some have suggested that it be studied as a potential chemotherapy. In fact, the Food and Drug Administration treats concentrated amounts of BBI like a drug.[12] Perhaps the most promising finding about BBI is that some studies have suggested that it may be one of the few agents with the ability to inactivate initiated cancer cells.[13] Remember, initiation is overwhelmingly irreversible.

Phytosterols

Phytosterols were discussed in Chapter 3. They have a structure that looks very much like cholesterol. This similarity seems to play a beneficial role. Phytosterols are so similar to cholesterol that they compete for absorption within the intestines. The end result is that less cholesterol gets absorbed.[14] In one large review of 80 studies on phytosterols, the authors concluded that the beneficial effects not only included lowering cholesterol but also in fighting

TABLE 7-2. PERCENTAGE OF PROTEASE INHIBITORS IN COOKED SOY FOODS VERSUS RAW SOY FLOUR

Food	Percent
Heated soy flour	4.3
Soy protein concentrates	8.9
Soy protein isolates	7.1
Textured vegetable protein (TVP)	5.0
Firm tofu	0.9
Tempeh burger	0.7
Soy breakfast strip	1.2
Soy breakfast patty	0.8
Wheat/soy pancake mix	4.5
Soymilk (dehydrated)	41.4
Frozen soymilk	0.4

SOURCES: DiPietro CM, Liener IE. Soybean protease inhibitors in foods. *J Food Sci.* 1989;54:606–617. Messina M, Messina V, Setchell K. *The Simple Soybean and Your Health.* Garden City Park, NY: Avery Publishing Group; 1994.

tumors.[15] This helps to support the observation that the Japanese and Seventh-Day Adventists who are vegetarian have the highest intake of phytosterols and the lowest rates of colon cancer.

Saponins

Saponins were also discussed in Chapter 3. They are glycosides—compounds made from sugars. Although they can be found in other legumes, the major dietary source is soy, which contains about 2% glycosides. No saponins come from animal proteins. Soy contains five kinds of saponins called soyasaponins.[16] Their role as anticarcinogens may be carried out through their antioxidant ability, which prevents oxygen free radicals from leading either to initiation or promotion.[17] But other studies have suggested that saponins are both directly and selectively toxic to certain cancer cells, regulate cell proliferation, and enhance our immune system.[18] All of these possibilities make soy saponins an interesting area of research for the future.

Phytates

Phytates are the plant storage form of phosphorus, a mineral that is necessary for every tissue in the body. Phytates are chelators, which means they bind in the intestines with minerals such as calcium and iron and help to carry them out of the body so they are not absorbed. At first this seems like a bad thing, and for a while phytates were in such disfavor that there was even an attempt to develop soybeans that were low in phytates.

However, like many other assumptions, things are not always as they appear. An increasing number of laboratory studies have shown that phytates inhibit colon cancer.[19] It seems that binding iron in our intestinal tract is the very reason why colon cancer is prevented and may even help prevent breast cancer. Iron is a large source of oxygen free radicals. But when it binds with phytates, the iron is no longer able to produce the free radicals. In one large review of 59 studies, it was concluded that it is not only the fiber in high-fiber diets, but also the phytates that protect us from breast and colon cancer.[20] Since excess amounts of iron have also been suggested to contribute to heart disease, including soy in your diet may be a simple way to help protect us.[21] Women in menopause would find this even more beneficial because they are no longer losing iron each month from menstruating.

Soy Anticarcinogens in Lesser Quantities

With the exception of the isoflavones that will be discussed next, the anticarcinogens above are the ones available in the greatest quantities in soy. However, several others exist. One class of organic compounds that contain only carbon and hydrogen and function as antioxidants is called terpenes. They are present in soy, but also in garlic, cereal grains, many vegetables, citrus fruits, and licorice root. Their role as antioxidants is believed to interrupt both initiation by cancer-causing agents and promotion by hormones. Another group of compounds found in soy that have antioxidant activity are the polyphenols. Like terpenes, they are also present in other foods, such as garlic, ginger, green tea, licorice root, broccoli, and others. Phenols are often used as disinfectants for the skin. Soy is also one of the few plants that is a source of omega-3 fatty acids, most commonly associated with fish, and capable of reducing the risk of both heart disease and cancer.

Isoflavones

Isoflavones are clearly the best studied of all of soy's anticarcinogens and are probably the main reason why soy is able to lower cancer risk. Of all the foods we are likely to eat, soy is the richest source of isoflavones. The two main isoflavones in soy are genistein and daidzein—both have a chemical structure similar to estrogen. But isoflavones have much weaker action, as little as one-hundred-thousandth as potent.[22]

Among the isoflavones, genistein is by far the most studied. Individual studies on genistein have shown that it is able to inhibit tyrosine kinase, a type of enzyme that oncogenes produce to stimulate the growth of cancer cells.[23] Genistein also inhibits angiogenesis, causing the slowing down of new blood vessel growth and making it more difficult for cancer cells to get the oxygen and nutrients they require to grow rapidly.[24] In addition to these steps that help to slow down cancer cell growth, genistein has the ability to reverse the changes a normal cell makes as it becomes undifferentiated—it actually causes cancer cells to

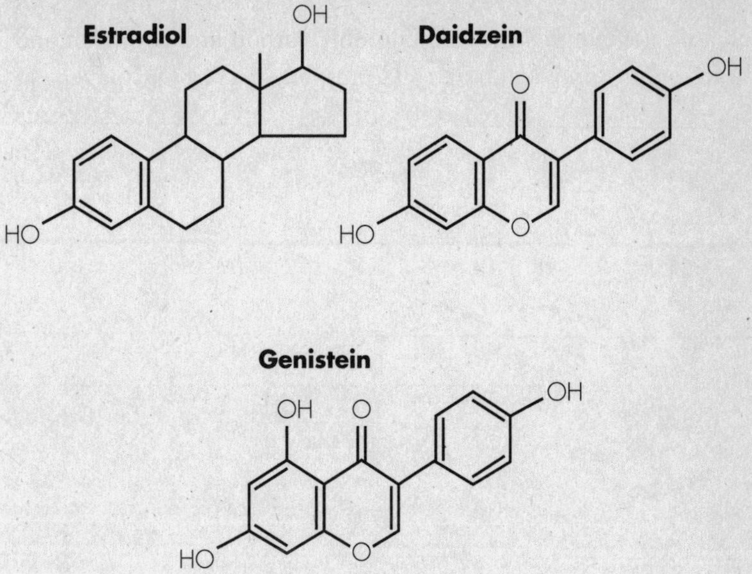

FIGURE 7-3.   Chemical Structure of Isoflavones

differentiate back to normal again.[25-27] Genistein is also a terrific source of antioxidants, which helps to prevent the changes in DNA that lead to cancer in the first place.[28, 29] There are now hundreds of scientific papers touting soy isoflavones as important allies in our personal fight to prevent cancer.

THE EVIDENCE FOR SOY IN RELATION TO SPECIFIC CANCERS

Every day, one person a minute in the United States dies of cancer. Despite all the advances in medicine, the numbers are growing. Imagine being able to harness all of the benefits of soy just by including soy in our diets. For women in menopause, only a handful of cancers account for a large percentage of the new diagnoses. I am going to explain what we know about how soy affects specific types of cancer.

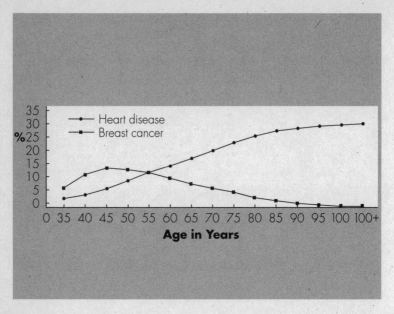

FIGURE 7-4. Deaths: Heart Disease versus Breast Cancer
SOURCE: National Center for Health Statistics: Vital Statistics of the
United States. Vol 11; 1990.

Breast Cancer

Although roughly 10 times more women will die of heart disease
than of breast cancer, survey after survey reveal that the majority
of women believe that they are more likely to die of breast cancer.

Not only is breast cancer life threatening, but surgery to cure
it may alter a woman's body in ways that are extremely damaging
to her self-esteem. There is little doubt that fear of getting breast
cancer is one of the main reasons that women look for an alternative to estrogen in the first place.

There is a strong association between a Western diet (high in
fat and protein and low in fiber and complex carbohydrates) and
breast cancer. In contrast, Japan has one of the lowest breast
cancer rates in the world. However, when Japanese women

TABLE 7-3. BREAST CANCER DEATH RATES 1994–1997

Country	Soy Intake (grams/day)	Death Rate/100,000
United States	Negligible	20
China	9.3	5
Japan	29.5	5.1

Source: Mortality Database 1994–1997, World Health Organization, 1999.

immigrate to the United States, their breast cancer rates approach the local population's, unless they maintain their Asian diet. These types of observations support the notion that it is diet and not genetics that protects these women from getting cancer.[30]

Because the Japanese diet is high in soy,[31] many believe that soy protects women from getting breast cancer. A number of epidemiological studies support this notion. For instance, in Singapore, women who ate more soy had lower breast cancer rates than those who ate less soy.[32] Chinese women who had high levels of isoflavones measured in their urine also were found to have a lower risk of breast cancer.[33] Both pre- and post-menopausal Asian-American women who continue to eat tofu have a lower rate of breast cancer than those who do not. In fact, those who eat it most often (greater than 120 times per year) have a 30% reduced risk.[34] And postmenopausal Australian women with breast cancer had lower 24-hour urine excretion of daidzein and genistein than postmenopausal woman without breast cancer studied for comparison.[35] Even animal studies suggest that a soy-based diet protects against breast cancer. Rats fed a diet of soy and then injected with chemicals known to cause breast cancer (dimethylbenz[α]anthracene and methylnitrosourea) were greatly protected from developing breast cancer.[36, 37] In a similar study, rats that were injected with a cancer-causing agent and fed a diet of soy protein isolate depleted of isoflavones developed less tumors and had a lower likelihood of developing breast cancer than rats who did not receive soy protein.[38]

In a slight twist on this experimental design, breast cancer cells were placed into a petri dish either with genistein or other substances and then injected into mice to see how many would develop breast cancer. It was found that pretreating the cancer cells with genistein lowered the cancer cell's ability to cause breast cancer in the mice. The same scientists placed human breast cancer cells into a petri dish with genistein and found that whether the breast cancer cells were estrogen receptor positive or negative, their growth was slowed down.[39] Other researchers have also found that genistein could slow the growth of both human and mouse cancer cells grown in petri dishes,[40–42] and combinations of genistein combined with daidzein and other soy isoflavones were found to be a potent inhibitor of cancer cell proliferation when added to breast cancer cells in a petri dish.[43] All of these studies and many similar ones in the scientific literature support a role for soy in breast cancer prevention.

Soy may also reduce breast cancer risk in a different way. Several studies have shown that a diet rich in soy is able to alter hormone levels significantly in premenopausal women by lowering their blood levels of the body's strongest estrogen, estradiol.[44] It is still not entirely clear how this happens, but it does not seem to be caused by an alteration of the hormones that stimulate estradiol production. Part of the reason for the lower estradiol levels seems to be caused by a change in its metabolism. Diets rich in isoflavones cause estradiol to become metabolized into 2-hydroxylated estrogens, a type of estrogen that is protective of breast cancer.[45] Because higher estrogen levels have been associated with an increased risk of breast cancer and because 2-hydroxyestrone is anticarcinogenic, soy may play an indirect preventive role in this fashion.

WHEN TO BEGIN

When is the best time to start eating soy if your goal is breast cancer protection? Should you begin at menopause, before, or after? The answer is we should start using soy in our diet before puberty.

As I mentioned in Chapter 2, a woman's breasts change throughout most of her life. The cells of breast tissue continue to mature from before puberty until well into adulthood. To explain this better, we need to take a closer look at the anatomy of a breast. Each breast contains 15 to 20 lobes, composed of groups of lobules: milk-producing glands. These lobules are connected together by breast tissue, blood vessels, and ducts. If we take an even closer look at each of the lobules we would find 10 to 100 rounded alveoli that open into the smallest branches of the milk ducts. These small branches join together to form larger ducts that end in the terminal or lactiferous ducts. Early in puberty, before ovulation and progesterone production begins, estrogen is just starting to be produced, but that amount of estrogen is enough to stimulate the ducts of the breasts to increase and branch (see Figure 2-1). A little later in puberty, ovulation begins and with it, the production of progesterone, which stimulates the alveolar cells to develop into lobules. Without progesterone, these changes do not occur.

When a girl enters her reproductive years, she develops regular menstrual cycles, causing the tips (called the terminal end buds) of the ducts, but not the bases, to divide more rapidly. Because the terminal end buds are the least mature terminal ductal structures, they are the ones most susceptible to carcinogens.[46] These terminal end buds are the growing fringes of the mammary gland, and they are undifferentiated. With each menstrual cycle, some of the terminal end buds mature (differentiate) as do the lobules. Remember, the more mature or differentiated a cell is, the more resistant it is to developing cancer.

Over time, the terminal end buds and lobules (which early in puberty before the first menstrual cycle are called type I lobules) become increasingly more differentiated. They progress to type II lobules. When women receive hormonal stimulation or become pregnant, they differentiate further to type III lobules. The most differentiated lobules, type IV, are only found in women who have been pregnant. This is why women who have had a full-term pregnancy early in life are four times less likely to develop breast cancer than women who never become pregnant.[47]

But for all of a woman's reproductive life until menopause, her breasts are in a constant state of change with each menstrual cycle—denser in the first half than in the second.[48] With each menstrual cycle, the cells of the breast divide, continuously becoming more mature (differentiated), and at the same time, at some potential risk for a carcinogen to cause a negative effect.

In laboratory studies, genistein has been given to immature rats to see how it affects breast development. The findings are interesting. When genistein is given before puberty, the rats' breasts have fewer terminal end buds and an increased number of type II lobules, both changes that make the breast less susceptible to chemical carcinogens (see Figure 7-5). In fact, when exposed to carcinogens after puberty these same rats were much more resistant to developing breast cancer than those who had not been fed genistein. The changes in breast development occurred after receiving genistein prepubertally, which may be an important part of why Asian women have a lower incidence of breast cancer.[49] In Singapore, 70% of children less than 10 years old have consumed soy products and of those more than 95% have consumed soy products before the age of 18 months.[50] Although soy-based infant formulas have been used in this country for more than 30 years, where isoflavones circulate at concentrations that are 13,000- to 22,000 times higher than plasma estradiol levels in early life,[51] it is too early to know if they will be helpful in lowering the risk of breast cancer. However, there may be an extraordinary opportunity for us to lower the risk of breast

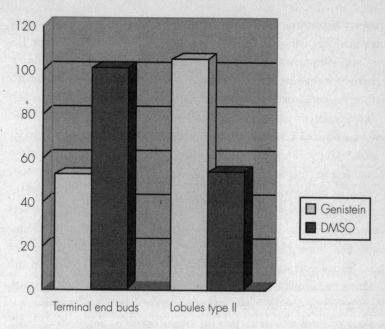

FIGURE 7-5.   Number of Mammary Terminal Ductal Structures in Female Rats Treated Prepubertally with Genistein or Dimethyl Sulfoxide (DMSO)

cancer in future generations of American women, by making soy available to our daughters before puberty.

THE CONFUSION SURROUNDING SOY AND BREAST CANCER

Why doesn't every menopausal woman choose soy over HRT? Some of the reasons have to do with not being used to the taste. Part of the reason has to do with the fact that most Western women interested in the benefits of soy usually start taking it before menopause instead of before puberty. There is less information about soy's effect on the breast if it is started later in life. I am a strong believer in getting started with soy whenever we become aware of its benefits. However, it is important to discuss some questions that have been raised about soy and breast health.

In one study, mice had their ovaries removed surgically to make them menopausal. At the same time, they were implanted with estrogen-dependent human breast cancer cells. Then the mice were fed either genistein or estradiol. The scientists found that the lowest dose of genistein made the cancer cells grow at a slow rate, much slower than the estradiol did.[52] Also, feeding the mice more than the lowest dose of genistein slowed the growth of the cancer cells. In another study, estrogen was used to stimulate estrogen-receptor-positive human breast cancer cells in a petri dish. The scientists found that adding a low dose of phytoestrogens caused a slight additional stimulation of the cancer cells, but just like the previous study, a higher dose of phytoestrogens slowed down the cancer cell growth in both estrogen-receptor-positive and the estrogen-receptor-negative cancer cells.[53] In another study, adding low doses of genistein to human breast cancer cells grown in cell culture and stimulated to grow with estrogen did not increase cancer cell proliferation any further. Adding a higher dose of genistein actually reduced the estradiol-stimulated cell proliferation.[54]

All these studies are difficult to interpret because they used cancer cells—cells that have already gone through initiation, promotion, and progression—and the studies were done in petri dishes, not in people. But what happens when women who do not have cancer eat soy? One study looked at premenopausal women with benign breast disease who were fed 60 grams of soy textured vegetable protein containing 45 milligrams (mg) of isoflavones for 2 weeks before they had a breast biopsy. The scientists studied 48 premenopausal women and reported that soy caused breast tissue cells to have an increase in their proliferation compared to breast tissue cells from women who did not get soy.[55]

However, the following year, another study of 84 premenopausal women taking identical amounts of soy for the same amount of time found that soy caused no increases in breast epithelial cell proliferation or any other measure of breast cell proliferation found in the previous study.[56] Even if there was some proliferation, that does not necessarily mean it would lead to breast cancer, because changes in breast epithelial cell proliferation routinely happens in women taking oral contraceptives containing either estrogen or estrogen and progesterone.[57] It is also important to remember that the breast is changing normally over the course of the menstrual cycle. It is more active in the second half of the cycle than in the first, and it is more active before menopause than after.[58] Responding to the hormonal changes of the menstrual cycle by proliferating is normal for breast cells.

THE BOTTOM LINE ON SOY AND BREAST CANCER

The overwhelming amount of information about soy supports a preventive role for breast cancer. Add to this the fact that no adverse effects of short- or long-term use of soy proteins are known in humans and it just makes sense to incorporate soy in our diets.[59] The greatest impact for breast cancer prevention might happen if we encourage the consumption of soy by girls before they reach puberty since that is what happens routinely in Asia. If we do, future generations of women in Western countries could see a decline in breast cancer.

But what about the majority of women who begin taking soy as an adult either before or after menopause? Is it both safe and protective? Once again, I believe the answer is yes. In addition to its direct benefits, consumption of soy diets containing isoflavones lower menstrual cycle estrogen and the adrenal hormone dehydroepiandrosterone sulfate (DHEA-S) and make menstrual cycle length longer, all things that are associated with lowering the risk of breast cancer.[60]

The best way to be sure you are getting the optimal amount is to consume amounts of soy comparable to the typical Asian diet. Try not to exceed 100 mg of isoflavones per day. More may be safe, but we do not have enough information to say for sure. You probably will get the best protection from eating soy foods, but if you do not like the taste or the texture, soy supplements may be the answer. One writer in the June 2001 issue of *Prevention* also believed soy to be a safe bet for breast protection but could not endorse soy nutritional supplements only because "of the risk of overdosing."[61] In my opinion, women are capable of taking the correct amount of a supplement as long as they are given the correct dosage information. That dose is ideally 50 mg per day and not more than 100 mg per day—within the range of the typical Asian diet.

The hardest question is whether or not women with breast cancer can safely take soy. No one is able to answer this question with certainty. Many people are unaware that there are a growing number of studies that show giving pharmaceutical estrogen to women with early stages of less aggressive breast cancer does not worsen their chances of survival.[62–64] Soy in tissue culture with breast cancer cells can cause some amount of stimulation—but always less than estrogen. Because quality of life must be considered along with extension of life, women with severe hot flashes or other significant menopausal symptoms should talk with their oncologists about the benefits and risks of taking soy for their particular situation. Do not be surprised if they say no. If they do, ask them why. Studies under way on the effect of soy and soy isoflavones at the University of North Carolina in women with advanced breast cancer and at the University of California at Los Angeles in patients with bilateral cancer recurrence who have had a mastectomy may shed further light on this question.

Soy and Uterine Cancer

Prevention of uterine cancer is one of the really exciting ways that soy may be useful. As with breast cancer, uterine cancer is seen much less often in countries where large amounts of soy are consumed.[65] Animal studies have shown that giving soy to rats made menopausal by removing their ovaries does not increase the weight of their uterus or stimulate the uterine lining.[66] Even more exciting, when soy isoflavones are added to primates treated with estrogen, estrogen is no longer able to cause proliferation of the uterine lining cells.[67]

All of this happens because soy acts just like the new class of medications called smart estrogens. Their real name is selective estrogen receptor modulators (SERMs). Soy is able to selectively promote bone and heart health while protecting against uterine cancer because it works primarily on the beta receptors of estrogen. We see similar effects in human studies. One report using soy extract corresponding to 50 mg of isoflavones daily showed no change in the growth of uterine lining cells.[68] Even a dose of 144 mg per day of soy extract did not affect the uterine lining cells.[69] As with the primate studies, adding conjugated equine estrogen to women taking soy isoflavones prevented the estrogen from causing proliferation changes in the uterine lining of the women studied.[70]

Soy is the perfect way to protect the uterine lining from the potential risks of estrogen. Soy itself does not stimulate the uterine lining, and it is also able to block the negative effects of estrogen. For these reasons, soy can be taken along with estrogen. A woman who still has her uterus must usually take progesterone along with estrogen to protect her uterine lining from being stimulated by estrogen. But progesterone may also cause some potentially harmful side effects (see Chapter 6). In the future, we may find that women who choose to take estrogen may be combining it with soy as an alternative to progesterone to get all the added benefits of soy with one less hormone pill to worry about.

Soy and Colon Cancer

Colon cancer is one of the most common causes of cancer deaths in the United States with 48,100 deaths and 98,200 new cases expected in 2001.[71] However, as with breast cancer and uterine cancer, the rates of colon cancer are lower in Asian countries where soy is routinely consumed than in countries where it is not.[72, 73] Certainly, people in Asian countries eat less animal protein, less fat, and more fiber. But even when these factors are taken into consideration, eating soy foods has been found to be protective against colon cancer. There are scientific reasons why soy is so well suited to lowering the risk of this potentially deadly disease.

Soy is believed to lower the risk of colon cancer because it is a source of a helpful bacteria in our intestines—bifidobacteria. What has this got to do with colon cancer? When you think of beans (including soybeans), one of the things that might come to mind is the fact that eating beans causes gas. That is because the bifidobacterium group and the 400 different kinds of bacteria, numbering in the trillions, in our colons[74] digest sugars that cannot be broken down by our digestive enzymes. They produce the gases carbon dioxide, hydrogen, and sometimes methane, which cause the flatulence for which beans are famous.[75] Soy helps to nurture the growth of bifidobacteria because two of the sugars that are abundant in soybeans—raffinose and stachyose— are particularly beneficial for bifidobacteria and of little use to most other bacteria in the colon.[76] When we eat soy, we are giving bifidobacteria a competitive edge, helping them to become plentiful in our intestinal tract.

This is good because bifidobacteria may have as one of its potential benefits the ability to prevent some types of cancers.[77] The higher the amount of bifidobacteria in the colon, the lower the amount of carcinogens in the feces.[78, 79] Dr. Messina points out in his book *The Simple Soybean and Your Health* that some health experts in Japan have even suggested replacing table sugar with sugars from soybeans to help promote the growth of bifidobacteria and reduce the risk of colon cancer. Fortunately, even small amounts of these sugars, less than it would take to cause flatulence and bloating, will increase the numbers of bifidobacteria in the intestine.[80] Because the bacteria in the body live in a delicate balance, eating a diet that includes soy may be particularly helpful because so many people take antibiotics. These are necessary medicines when harmful bacteria threaten our lives. But overuse of antibiotics may lead to a reduction in some of the helpful bacteria in our colon that protect us from certain types of cancer and may explain the increased amounts of certain cancers seen in people who take too many antibiotics.

The nutritional content of soy may also help reduce the risk of colon cancer. You are aware that fiber lowers the risk of colon cancer, and you probably know that eating fruits and vegetables also lowers the risk. Two important nutritional factors found in soy also help keep colon cancer away—folic acid and calcium.[81, 82] Eating soy is a terrific way to help ensure you get enough of this important vitamin and mineral.

Soy contains the phytoestrogens genistein and daidzein, which contribute to its ability to protect against colon cancer. Did you know that estrogen has a protective role on the colon?[83, 84] There are roughly the same numbers of estrogen receptors on normal colon cells as there are on normal breast cells.[85] Women who take estrogen replacement therapy are less likely to die from colon cancer than those who do not,[86] and treatment with the antiestrogen tamoxifen may increase the risk of colon cancer.[87] The fact that the concentrations of soy isoflavones are extremely high in the colons of people who consume soy regularly, especially if they are vegetarians, has caused the belief that they are protective to the cells that line the colon.[88] In animal studies done with rodents, phytoestrogens found in both linseed, which is rich in lignans, and in soy (genistein) as well as soy itself slow the rate of cancer cells in the colon and appeared to lower the risk of getting colon cancer.[89–91] Although more studies need to be done in humans to prove conclusively that soy reduces colon cancer risk, the evidence in favor of soy is mounting. This is one more reason to include it in our diets.

Soy and Prostate Cancer

Many women who read this book have male family members or friends in the age range when prostate cancer is diagnosed. Sixty percent of men over the age of 60 will have cancer cells in their prostate. According to the American Cancer Society, men in the United States were diagnosed with 180,400 new cases of prostate cancer in 2000, and 31,900 deaths—almost the identical numbers to the comparable information on breast cancer in women (182,800 and 40,800 respectively).[92] For this reason, I will discuss the importance of soy in preventing men from dying of prostate cancer.

In Japan and some other Asian countries, the number of men with prostate cancer is roughly the same—but there is one important difference. The prostate cancers remain small and do not spread. Far fewer men in Asia die from this disease.[93–95] Dr. Herman Adlercreutz, one of the leading scientists in the world involved in soy research, believes the answer is the isoflavones found in soy. Hundreds of studies have provided both animal data and studies of human prostate cancer cells that show soy isoflavones slow the growth of prostate cancer cells.[96–99] Evidence shows that men, as well as women, should include soy in their diets.

Soy and Other Cancers

Soy and soy isoflavones may prove to have beneficial effects on other cancers as well. These include cancers of the head and neck;[100] solid pediatric tumors such as neuroblastomas; as well as leukemia, melanoma, rhabdomyosarcomas, Ewing's sarcomas, and others. The ability to slow down new blood vessel growth and many other anticarcinogenic abilities make soy an important part of everyone's diet.

chapter 8

OTHER HEALTH BENEFITS OF SOY

Soy is a terrific example of a food that blurs the distinction between conventional and medicinal or functional foods.[1] Soy is a superb source of high-quality protein and is considered a useful aid in the prevention and treatment of chronic disease. Let's talk about some other health benefits of soy.

DIABETES

Diabetes affects between 6 and 7 percent of the American population—about 16 million people. Unfortunately, one third of these do not realize they have the disease. Estimates place the number of new cases each year at 800,000 and unless things change dramatically, the total number of people with diabetes will climb to 23 million in just 10 years.[2]

Diabetes is an equal opportunity disease. It spares no ages and no ethnic or racial background. According to the most recent figures, it kills roughly 200,000 Americans, depriving them of 2 million years of life because on average diabetes shortens the average life expectancy by as much as 15 years.[3] Diabetes is the leading cause of kidney failure (nephropathy), blindness in adults (retinopathy), and leg and foot amputations. Diabetes is also a major risk factor for heart disease (2 to 4 times those of people without diabetes), stroke (high blood pressure affects over 60%), and birth defects (3 to 4 times those of nondiabetics). The nerve damage caused by diabetes can also lead to impotence. At present diabetes has no cure. Each year the United States spends over $100 billion in health-related expenditures—$1 of every $10 of health-care dollars and $1 of every $4 of Medicare dollars.

Risk Factors for Diabetes

- Positive family history
- Obesity
- Decreased physical activity
- Western lifestyle

What Is Diabetes?

Diabetes has been around a long time. A description of the disease was first recorded on Egyptian papyrus around 1500 B.C. However, it took until A.D. 100 for Greek physicians to name it. Diabetes means "siphon," probably because one of the most common symptoms is increased urination. Doctors noticed that ants were attracted to the urine of diabetic patients. Around 1650, a British physician named Thomas Willis tasted the urine of one of his patients and found it to be "wondrous sweet." The sweetness of the urine caused the name to be changed to diabetes mellitus, or "honey siphon." Around the close of the nineteenth century, classic experiments by J. Von Mering and Oskar Minkowski proved that diabetes was caused by a deficiency in the pancreas.[4] They found that by removing the pancreas from a dog it developed diabetes. But it took until 1921–1922 for Doctors Fred Banting, Charles Best, and John Collip to identify and produce the hormone made deficient by removing the pancreas. That hormone became known as insulin.[5]

We now know that diabetes is not a single disease, but a group of disorders that share certain common features—the main one is elevated levels of blood glucose. Normally when we eat, our digestive tract breaks down complex carbohydrates into glucose. The glucose is absorbed into our bloodstream and becomes our blood sugar. But in order for our cells to use glucose as fuel, it has to get into the cell. That is where insulin comes into play. Insulin is stored in the beta cells of the pancreas. When blood glucose levels rise, the pancreas secretes insulin, which attaches to the surface of cells and allows the glucose to enter and be broken down for fuel. Without enough insulin, the cells starve, blood glucose levels rise, and the medical problems associated with diabetes begin. There are two common types of diabetes—Type 1 and Type 2.

Type 1 diabetes used to be called insulin-dependent diabetes mellitus, or IDDM. It is caused by an autoimmune destruction of the insulin-producing beta cells. The body literally turns against its own beta cells and destroys them. Eventually, the person with Type 1 diabetes no longer makes insulin and must take an injection of it daily. Without insulin a person with Type 1 diabetes would die.

This type of diabetes usually begins in childhood or early adulthood, so it used to be called juvenile-onset diabetes, but we now know it can occur at any age. There are about 1 million people with Type 1 diabetes and over 13,000 new cases are diagnosed each year. Although Type 1 diabetes is the smaller group, people who have this disease must live with it for most of their lifetime. Therefore, they have more time to develop many of the problems it causes.

Type 2 diabetes used to be called non-insulin-dependent diabetes mellitus, or NIDDM. Because it occurs more commonly after the age of 40, it has also been called adult-onset diabetes. It currently affects about 15 million people. Most Type 2 diabetics can control their elevated glucose levels with either a healthful diet, exercise, and/or oral medications called oral hypoglycemic agents. However, about 2.5 million need to take insulin to keep their blood glucose levels in the normal range. Unfortunately, Type 2 diabetes is becoming increasingly common in younger people, even in childhood, especially in minority populations. Genes are in part responsible for Type 2 diabetes, but they are different genes than the ones responsible for Type 1 diabetes. Some of the reasons we are seeing more of this disease has to do with poor dietary habits, too little exercise, and an alarming rate of obesity. Approximately 55% of the adult population in the United States is overweight, of which 22% are obese. That translates into over 97 million American adults.

Type 2 diabetes is complicated, because two problems are going on at the same time. One is that the cells of the body become resistant to insulin. An increased amount of fat cells adds to the insulin resistance. About 80% to 90% of diabetics are overweight. Most of the fat is in the belly—the so-called apple shape rather than pear shape. The second problem is that although the pancreas tries to deliver the correct amount of insulin in response to glucose, the pattern of release and the amount secreted are not enough to overcome the insulin resistance. Sometimes the oral hypoglycemic agents or insulin cause the blood sugar to fall too low, which causes hypoglycemia, which can be dangerous and lead to life-threatening convulsions. As you can see, controlling blood glucose levels within the normal range is the only way a person with diabetes can prolong life and reduce the risk of long-term complications.

How Diet Affects Diabetes

Doctors have known for a long time that diet affects the health of people with diabetes. In Egyptian times, doctors prescribed "wheat, fresh grits, grapes, honey, berries, and sweet beer." Later the Greeks added to the Egyptian recommendations by including sweet wine and milk. However, this view of diet changed radically by the eighteenth century as doctors switched their beliefs and thought carbohydrates were absolutely to be avoided.[6] Avoidance of carbohydrates persisted for another two centuries until the medical community took notice that in cultures where diabetes was rare, the people's diet was based largely on the complex carbohydrates found in plant foods. Also in those cultures, obesity is extremely rare and the percentage of their calories coming from fat is low—sometimes less than 10%.

Soy is low in saturated fat and contains no cholesterol, which is important because people with diabetes are at increased risk for atherosclerosis. A vegetarian diet that consists of soy also contributes to weight loss. In one study of 208 postmenopausal women aged 45 to 74, those who consumed a high amount of genistein had a significantly lower body mass index (BMI), waist circumference, and fasting insulin level than those women who did not eat genistein. Animal studies in rodents also show that genetically obese mice fed a diet of soy protein isolate lose body fat significantly more than mice fed milk whey protein.[7] A low-fat diet can be beneficial for controlling blood glucose levels.[8]

Soy and Diabetes

One of the early advocates for soy as an excellent source of food for people with diabetes came in the early 1900s from Dr. John Harvey Kellogg of the corn flakes fame. In his sanatorium in Battle Creek, Michigan, Dr. Kellogg recommended his diabetic patients eat soy foods and other vegetables. About the same time, two doctors named Friedenwald and Ruhrah found that if their diabetic patients ate soy, they had less sugar in their urine, which is a measure of diabetes control.[9] Some of the dietary benefits of soy on diabetes can be explained by the discovery, in 1981, of the glycemic index.[10] Different foods have a different effect on blood glucose levels. The scientists fed healthy fasting volunteers 62 common foods and measured their blood glucose levels over the next 2 hours. Glucose—ordinary sugar—produces a blood sugar response rated at 100%. The glycemic index of soybeans was 10% to 20%. Brown rice, by comparison, has a 60% to 69% rating.

The glycemic index was a way to quantify that legumes such

as soybeans were digested slowly, causing blood glucose to rise in a slow, steady rise rather than quickly as a sharp spike that stressed the pancreas to produce insulin quickly and in large amounts. Soy differs from many other legumes in that it does not contain a significant amount of starch.[11] Soy fiber can reduce the amount of insulin released from the pancreas when people with Type 2 diabetes who have high cholesterol are fed a large dose of glucose.[12] This is very important because it puts less immediate demand on the person's pancreas.

Soy can also be valuable in preventing blood glucose levels from dropping too low. Some people have a condition known as reactive hypoglycemia. After a meal, the person's pancreas responds too briskly causing the blood glucose levels to drop uncomfortably low. This causes the person to feel dizzy, tired, and cranky. By smoothing out the release of insulin, soy helps to keep blood glucose levels closer to the normal range without wide fluctuations that are too high or too low. All of this helps people with diabetes maintain better blood sugar control.

KIDNEY DISEASES

Our kidneys are two very busy filters, cleansing some 45 gallons of blood every day, keeping in our bloodstream the nutrients that we need while allowing waste or unwanted material to pass out into the urine. When our kidneys become affected by disease, the toxic substances in our bloodstream accumulate. Because kidney disease is a progressive problem, it can become very serious, and the toxic substances can eventually lead to our death.

In Chapter 3, we discuss that too much animal protein overworks our kidneys, especially if we have kidney disease. The more the kidneys have to filter (called an increased glomerular filtration rate, or GFR), the harder they have to work and the more vulnerable they become to disease. Some authorities believe that a low-protein diet, especially one that includes soy, could even slow down the rate of kidney disease in people with diabetes. Here is why.

TABLE 8-1. EFFECT OF PROTEIN TYPE ON GLOMERULAR FILTRATION RATE (GFR)

Protein	Percent Increase in GFR
Beef	50
Chicken	35
Fish	20
Soy	None

In one Italian study, patients with kidney disease who were fed a diet of soy protein for 2 months had a 16% lower glomerular filtration rate than when they ate a diet of animal protein.[13] These same researchers 1 year later fed a soy protein diet to volunteers with kidney disease for 4 months and found that they lost significantly less protein in their urine over the entire period of time.[14] In addition, their blood cholesterol levels came down. This shows the enormous benefit that soy provides our kidneys, especially if kidney disease is present.

Kidney Stones

About 10% of men and 3% of women will have a kidney stone sometime during their adult life. It is considered one of the most painful experiences to endure. About 80% of all stones are made of calcium oxalate, either alone or with a nucleus of calcium phosphate or calcium apatite.[15] In one large study, 45,619 men between the ages of 40 and 70 who never had a kidney stone were followed for 4 years. Intake of animal protein was directly associated with the risk of kidney stone formation. The more they ate, the greater the chance they had of developing a kidney stone.[16] In another report, British vegetarians who consumed a low-protein diet were half as likely to form kidney stones as people in the general population.[17] These findings occur because animal protein causes more calcium to be excreted in the kidneys than does plant protein. This happens in part because soy has less sulfur-containing amino acids compared with animal protein. The increased sulfur in the urine encourages the kidneys to excrete calcium. As the urine becomes more saturated with calcium, crystals form that attach to the cells of the kidney, forming the beginning of a stone. Another reason that soy may reduce the risk of kidney stones is that the fiber in it binds calcium in the intestinal tract, preventing some of the calcium from being absorbed. Reducing the risk of kidney stones is one more reason to incorporate soy into our diets.

GALLSTONES

The gallbladder is a sac about the size of the ball of your thumb. It is located just beneath the liver. It secretes bile into the digestive tract, which helps digest fats. Bile is made of cholesterol, bile acids, lecithin, and water within the gallbladder. Cholesterol cannot dissolve in the water, so it must be incorporated into a mixture with lecithin and bile salts. If the amount of cholesterol increases or the amount of bile acids, lecithin, or water decreases, cholesterol precipitates and a stone forms. Gallstones are a common problem in perimenopausal and menopausal women who are overweight.[18] They are another example of a problem caused by a Western diet. Gallstones can be made purely of cholesterol, or cholesterol mixed with bile pigments and calcium salts, or they can be made entirely of minerals or a pure pigment (calcium bilirubinate). About 80% of the gallstones found in people in the United States are the mixed type; most of the remaining 20% are made purely of minerals.

Many studies have shown that a diet rich in fiber can reduce the incidence of gallstones.[19] One study in Italy of 15,910 men and 13,674 women found a high-fiber intake a very significant predictor of women who would not develop gallstones.[20] Women with gallstones are more likely to consume higher amounts of total fats, monounsaturated fatty acids, saturated fatty acids, and cholesterol.[21] Soy is a rich source of fiber, extremely low in saturated fats, and contains no cholesterol. It also contains lecithin, an essential component of bile. In animal studies, rodents fed a soybean diet had the lowest levels of cholesterol in their bile.[22]

Similarly, both buckwheat protein and soy protein reduce gallstone formation in hamsters,[23] and soy protein has actually helped to dissolve gallstones after they were formed.[24] The more soy you include in your diet, the less likely you are to get gallstones.

SOY AND HIGH BLOOD PRESSURE

High blood pressure (hypertension) is a strong and independent risk factor for heart disease. Hypertension affects roughly 60 million Americans. That translates into 20.3% of American women ages 20 to 74.[25, 26] People with hypertension do not have any symptoms, so nearly one third either do not know they have it or they stop taking their medications to treat it. Of course, that is a big mistake because hypertension left untreated can lead to heart problems, stroke, and kidney failure. This is why it is called the "silent killer."

There are some simple things we can do to make high blood pressure lower. One definite preventive measure is to bring on the vegetables. In addition to soy, vegetarian diets lower blood pressure.[27, 28] In these and many other reports, a vegetarian diet not only lowers blood pressure but also helps the patients who were being studied improve their exercise tolerance, if they have a history of heart disease or stroke. Soy may be of particular benefit in lowering blood pressure.

Something in soybeans may act like the drugs called angiotensin-converting enzyme (ACE) inhibitors. These drugs are widely used and act by inhibiting the body's production of angiotensin, an enzyme that causes blood vessels to constrict. A group of Japanese scientists isolated an ACE-inhibiting enzyme out of soy sauce and found that it could lower blood pressure in hypertensive rats. Before you start dousing your food with soy sauce, remember it contains a lot of salt that can make your hypertension worse. The point is, there seems to be something in soy sauce or soy in general that lowers blood pressure in a specific way.

Another theory of how soy helps to lower blood pressure has to do with its lower level of sulfur-containing amino acids compared with animal proteins. Diets high in protein, but particularly in animal protein, cause the body to retain sodium. This makes the body work harder to break down and excrete the byproducts of the sulfur amino acids. The more sodium that is retained, the more likely it is to lead to fluid retention and ultimately to hypertension. Because soy contains lower levels of sulfur amino acids, it allows more sodium to be excreted in the urine and in part may account for the reduced blood pressure found in vegetarians.[29]

Look at the animal data related to soy and lower blood pressure. Rodents are commonly used as animal models for this purpose. In one study, mice with high blood pressure were fed a diet high in salt to make their blood pressure even higher. When soy was also added to the diet, their blood pressure values lowered.[30] Mice with naturally occurring high blood pressure have also been studied. Feeding them a diet of soy protein lowered their blood pressure. There are a large number of studies showing soy's effectiveness in lowering blood pressure in hypertensive mice.

Other than the epidemiological studies in vegetarians that I mentioned above, there are only a few studies of soy's effect on blood pressure in humans. One group of scientists studied people with high-normal blood pressure values and did not see a lowering of blood pressure.[31] However, another study in 51 perimenopausal women with normal blood pressures given a soy dietary supplement twice daily did have a significant decrease in their diastolic blood pressure (the denominator, or bottom number, of the blood pressure fraction).[32] We have to remember that in both of these studies, the people who were studied had either high-normal or normal blood pressure. Until more studies are done using only soy to treat high blood pressure, we will not know for certain how effective it is. But we can say that eating soy along with other vegetables is a lot better for your blood pressure than eating animal protein.

In addition to a potential role in high blood pressure, soy may play an important role in keeping our heart's blood vessel walls free of plaque and helping them to remain elastic (see Chapter 6). Menopausal monkeys fed soy containing isoflavones had significantly less plaque form in their coronary arteries (the ones that bring blood to the heart) than monkeys fed soy with its isoflavones removed.[33] They also found that blood vessels remained more elastic in monkeys fed soy—just as elastic as those given estrogen and even more elastic than those given estrogen plus medroxyprogesterone acetate.[34]

Studies in humans show that soy offers similar benefits.[35] The arteries in 21 women aged 46 to 67 who took soy isoflavones (80 mg per day for 5 to 10 weeks) were 26% more elastic than the arteries in women who took a placebo.[36] These findings are nearly identical to what happens when postmenopausal women are treated with long-term estrogen replacement therapy (ERT).[37] Soy is a terrific food to help you maintain a healthy cardiovascular system.

LACTOSE INTOLERANCE

Lactose intolerance affects hundreds of millions of people worldwide.[38] It affects 70% to 90% of Asian, black, Native American, and Mediterranean adults and 10% to 15% of northern and western Europeans. It is due to a deficiency of the enzyme lactase, which is usually located in the cells of the small intestine. When there is not enough lactase, a person cannot digest the most common sugar in milk—lactose. The undigested lactose passes through the digestive tract to the colon, and bacteria there ferment the sugar, which produces gases and organic acids. The end result is bloating, abdominal pain, gas, and sometimes, explosive, watery diarrhea.

Fortunately, most babies have always been able to digest lactose. Lactose is the main sugar in cow's milk and in mother's milk. Many children lose their lactase enzyme sometime between 3 and 7 years of age. Some babies do not tolerate cow's milk. Soy formulas are widely used for feeding babies with cow-milk allergy.[39] Adults with cow-milk allergy find soymilk an excellent substitute as well, because it contains no lactose and no cow-milk protein. This is just one more health benefit provided by this magnificent bean.

STRENGTH TRAINING

When we think of trying to bulk up for the Olympics, eating a tasty meal of soy might not be the first thing that comes to your mind. Think again! In a study of 66 Romanian Olympic endurance athletes training for kayak-canoe and rowing, half were fed soy protein (1½ grams per kilogram, which is a large amount) for 8 weeks and the other half ate their typical foods with no soy protein. They worked and trained for 4 to 6 hours daily. After 2 months, the group that ate the soy protein gained 3 kilograms (6.6 pounds) of mostly lean body mass; increased their strength indexes, blood count, and total calcium; and had a significant decrease of fatigue after training compared to the other group of athletes. Based on these findings, the study supported soy protein as a beneficial option for the preparation of top endurance athletes.[40] Whether you are eating for health, nutrition, enjoyment, or exercise, think soy!

chapter 9

OTHER NON-ESTROGEN APPROACHES TO MENOPAUSE

Choices for the treatment of menopause and its symptoms are neither new nor limited to estrogen and soy. In fact, if we look back to the 1899 *Merck Manual,* recommendations included ammonia, black cohosh, camphor, cannabis indica (marijuana), change of air, eucalyptus, hot springs, opium, and suc ovarian (the juice from cow ovaries crushed up at the slaughterhouse). Over the past century we have kept one or two choices from that list (such as black cohosh), eliminated most of the rest, and added quite a few more including some unconventional steroids and a whole lot of herbs and supplements.

Not everything being used is "natural," "safe," and "gentle." A number of the products marketed as natural botanicals come from plants—only they are chemical plants. Some work, some do not. Some should not be taken with other medications; some are just plain risky. But before reviewing the herbs themselves, I want to discuss how widely herbs and alternative medicines are used.

HOW WIDELY ARE HERBS AND ALTERNATIVE MEDICINE USED?

Alternative approaches to menopause are so widely used I'm beginning to wonder why they are the choices that are called alternative. Let us review some information from a telephone survey conducted between April 27 and May 16, 1999, by *Prevention* magazine and Princeton Survey Research Associates of a nationally representative sampling of 2,000 adults (margin of error ± 2%). The information is not limited to menopause, but the results tell us a lot about the use of dietary supplements in the United States.

According to the *Prevention* survey, the number of adults in the age group 45 to 64 will grow 51% by the year 2010. These numbers have a real impact on health-care dollars because health-care expenditures increase 39% when the head of household turns 55. According to *Prevention,* 47% of consumers think their health plan is more concerned about making money than providing care. That is probably why the consumers who use dietary supplements classified themselves as a self-care group, not an alternative care or supplement group. The following statistics support their view:

Use of Herbal Remedies

- 49% (91,147,209) used an herbal remedy within the past 12 months
- 45% (74,400,000) are more likely to treat themselves first
- 24% (44,643,531) regularly use an herbal remedy

Common Reasons for Using Herbal Remedies

- 75% ensure good health
- 61% improve energy

- 58% prevent/treat colds
- 43% improve memory
- 41% reduce anxiety
- 35% ease depression
- 29% prevent/treat serious illness

How Consumers Use Herbal Remedies

- 36% instead of prescriptions
- 31% with prescriptions
- 48% instead of over-the-counter (OTC) products
- 30% with OTC products

Reasons for Using Herbal Remedies Instead of Prescriptions

- 43% prefer natural/organic products
- 21% fewer side effects
- 14% more effective
- 11% allow me to treat myself
- 8% less expensive
- 6% more gentle/mild

The *Prevention* survey also found out where consumers learn about dietary supplements:

- 51% friends/family
- 43% magazines
- 41% product labels
- 39% advertising
- 38% books
- 28% doctor
- 28% health food stores
- 23% pharmacist

- 19% alternative medicine practitioner
- 13% Internet
- 10% 1-800 number

These statistics tell us that people who self-care also self-educate. This is why it is important to have reliable information available—little decision-making is directed by the medical community, and they often learn from the same sources their patients do.

In a more recent survey with a focus on menopause, Nora Keenan of the Centers for Disease Control and Prevention added to what we learned from the *Prevention* survey. She told an audience at the National Institutes of Health (NIH) on October 27, 2000, that nearly half of menopausal women are using complementary medicine therapies including vitamins, herbs, and soy to help them treat their symptoms.

About 2,600 women age 45 to 98 (median age 60) were surveyed by state officials in Florida, Tennessee, and Minnesota. Of those, 44% had reached natural menopause and another 39% were menopausal due to surgery. Only 17% of the women surveyed were still menstruating.

The survey found that 21% used complementary or alternative therapies alone, and 25% used both conventional and alternative methods. Taken together, that was more than twice the 19% who said they used conventional medications such as estrogen. The most popular therapies were vitamins and minerals followed by herbal remedies, with soy, mind/body programs, acupuncture, and related techniques following after the herbs. Roughly one third of all the women said they did not use any therapy to treat their symptoms.

With all the talk about estrogen, it is interesting that more than twice the number of women prefer complementary and alternative approaches to traditional options for treating their menopausal symptoms. But a stroll through your supermarket, pharmacy, or health food store will reveal incredible numbers of vitamins, minerals, and herbs lining the shelves. Nearly 100 million American adults—over 40% of the nation's adult population—are buying them. It was estimated that in 1998, each U.S. health food store sold over half a million dollars' worth of herbs alone, and that does not include vitamins and other dietary supplements.[1] That translated into more than $6 billion worth of dietary supplements in 1998[2] and a dietary supplement industry that in 2001 is likely to exceed $12 billion in the United States alone.[3]

As pointed out, the people who used these herbs are not necessarily against prescription medicines. In fact 15 million U.S. adults take their herbals right along with their prescription medicines; half of all patients do not mention their herbal remedies to their physicians, sometimes even when they are asked. I think this reluctance stems from patients' concerns that their doctors will disapprove.

If that happens, you have the wrong doctor. Slowly but steadily the traditional American doctors are becoming open to herbal remedies.[4] In fact, 4% of all vitamins, minerals, and

TABLE 9-1. GLOBAL SUPPLEMENT MARKET 1999 (MARKET VOLUME: U.S. $46 BILLION)

	VMS	Herbal/Homeopathy	Sport/Specialty	Total
North America	7.1	4.0	3.4	14.5
Europe	3.7	6.7	1.9	12.3
Asia	1.5	5.1	1.0	7.6
Japan	3.5	2.2	1.4	7.1
Rest of world	2.0	1.4	1.1	4.5
Total	17.8	19.4	8.8	46.0

NOTE: In retail prices.
VMS = vitamins/minerals/supplements
SOURCE: Gruenwald J, Nutraceuticals World. July/August 2000;36.

herbal supplements in the United States, to the tune of $400 million, are being purchased from American practitioners. Consumers made 44% of those purchases from chiropractors, 33% from medical doctors (mostly general and family practitioners), 3% from physicians' assistants, 1% from nurses, and 19% from various alternative practitioners.[5] In Europe the percentages are even higher—the majority of European doctors embrace alternative approaches to menopause. In Germany, for instance, doctors overwhelmingly embrace herbs—70% of German general practitioners prescribe herbal remedies. Over there, St. John's wort outsells Prozac 8 to 1.

Of course vitamins, minerals, and herbal supplements are not the only alternative medicine that Americans use. As recently as 1993, David Eisenberg and his colleagues at Harvard Medical School documented that many Americans use both traditional practitioners and alternative practitioners, and an increasing number prefer alternative practitioners.[6] The total visits to alternative medicine practitioners jumped 47% from 427 million in 1990 to 629 million in 1997, many more than the 386 million trips to primary-care doctors during the same period. Eisenberg also found that 4 out of 10 Americans paid an estimated $21.2 billion for alternative services including herbal medicine, megavitamins, homeopathy, chiropractic, and acupuncture. Most of the users of alternative medicine, 58%, are attempting to prevent illness or enhance health maintenance. The remaining 42% used it to treat existing illness. Both of these categories are important to menopausal women.

CURRENT REGULATION OF HERBS
IN THE UNITED STATES

Prevention magazine, in its 1999 survey, asked if the federal government regulates supplements to ensure safety. The results may surprise you—16% of the participants did not know, 50% thought no, and 34% thought the answer was yes. Obviously, the American public is confused about the regulation of herbal products. Some of the confusion may be because the degree of regulation in the United States has changed over time and varies across the world. Herbal products are seen as drugs in several countries, for example in Germany, France, and Scandinavia, while the same products are freely available in the United Kingdom and the Netherlands.

The regulatory policies of the United States evolved over about 100 years (see Table 9-2). We inherited a large knowledge base about herbs from Europe, and early Americans used many Native American Indian plant medicines. But many of these herbal remedies were abandoned because of misuse, overconfident expectations, and outright fraudulent advertising by the makers of patented medicine. Two things resulted from the patent medicine scams: (1) The Food and Drug Administration (FDA) was developed along with laws that require a drug to be safe and effective, and (2) laws were developed that prevented patenting of anything from nature.

As a result, American manufacturers shunned herbals and became experts at using high-tech drug development to produce medications, which they were allowed to patent and sell for a good profit. Herbals fell to the wayside because studies necessary to satisfy the FDA's standards for safety and effectiveness take on average 12 years and cost up to $300 to $800 million—too high a cost for companies to make a profit on an OTC medicine. This is why most of what we read about herbals comes from epidemiological observations of safe use for a long time in Europe and Asia or studies done in other parts of the world. We are just beginning to produce good clinical trials involving the use of herbal remedies in the United States, but the number and the substances studied are still limited. See Table 9-2 for a quick chronology of government regulation of herbs.

TABLE 9-2. REGULATION OF HERBS—A BRIEF HISTORY

1906	Food and Drug Act	Prohibited the shipment of "adulterated" or "misbranded" drugs across state lines
1912	Sherley Amendment	Prohibited fraudulent claims on a label
1938	Federal Food, Drug and Cosmetic Act	Required testing for safety before marketing a new drug. Most botanicals were exempt from testing
1962	Kefauver-Harris Amendment	Required drugs marketed thereafter be proven effective as well as safe; exempted drugs marketed prior to 1938
1972	Kefauver-Harris Amendment expanded	17 panels created (one for each different therapeutic class of drugs, i.e., analgesics, laxatives, etc.) to examine the active ingredients of OTC drugs. Majority of herbal drugs classified as OTC. Established that the created panels would decide if botanicals could continue to be marketed or removed from the market if their claims for effectiveness could not be proven. Conducted no studies, relied on existing ones
1990	OTC panel reports issued	Category I—generally recognized as safe and effective, and not misbranded. Category II—not generally recognized as safe and effective, or misbranded (included the majority, even prune juice concentrate, because no clinical data were available on its effectiveness as a laxative). Category III—insufficient data
1994	Dietary Supplement Health and Education Act	Defines a dietary supplement as any product (besides tobacco) that contains a vitamin, mineral, herb, or amino acid that is intended to supplement the normal diet

SOURCE: Modified from Israelsen LD, Blumenthal M. FDA issues final rules for structure/function claims for dietary supplements under DSHEA. *HerbalGram*. 2000;48:32–38.

The Dietary Supplement Health and Education Act of 1994

The Dietary Supplement Health and Education Act (DSHEA) came into existence in October of 1994, and it was a direct result of the American public generating more calls, letters, and faxes of support to Congress for this bill than any other bill to that time. The public made it clear that the OTC panel reports were depriving them of dietary supplements, and they wanted and demanded the right to maintain an individual's right to self-medicate. You might have guessed from the term "dietary supplement" that under the provisions of DSHEA the FDA considers supplements to be foods and not drugs. Like foods, dietary supplements are ingested (either as a pill, capsule, tablet, or liquid), but they cannot be represented as conventional food or the sole item of a meal or diet. In addition, dietary supplements must be labeled as a supplement.

Supplements may be marketed without testing for effectiveness, proof of safety, or proof of marketing claims, as long as (here is the catch) they make no claim to diagnose, treat, cure, or prevent disease. This is different from OTC drugs (such as pain or cold remedies) and prescription drugs that need to be proven safe and effective by manufacturers before they are approved. A dietary supplement is considered unsafe if:

- It presents a significant risk of illness or injury with ordinary use
- No conditions of use are recommended on the label
- There is a new dietary ingredient that has inadequate safety information
- It contains an ingredient that renders it adulterated

If a significant safety concern is raised about a supplement, the Secretary of Health and Human Services may declare an imminent hazard and stop the supplement from being sold after giving the manufacturer a 10-day written notice. The DSHEA also created (1) a Commission of Dietary Supplement Labels to recommend regulations of all claims and statements made about dietary supplements and (2) the Office of Dietary Supplements within the National Institutes of Health to promote the scientific study of the usefulness of dietary supplements.

The public wanted the right to self-medicate. Now they are worried they also got the right to self-regulate. In the meantime, they are in the process of trying to self-educate. The FDA does have very clear regulations in place, but they are far from perfect. No wonder there is concern and confusion. If you are interested in the full text of the DSHEA and have access to the Internet, you can get it at *www.fda.gov/OHRMS/DOCKETS/98fr/oc99257.pdf*.

STRUCTURE/FUNCTION STATEMENTS

Before the DSHEA was passed, all health claims on supplements had to be approved by the FDA just as they are for food. Since the DSHEA was passed, things have changed. That is the role of structure/function statements. Look at almost any bottle or box of a nutritional supplement and you will see phrases describing what that particular supplement is supposed to do. The FDA does not have to approve these claims, but the manufacturers have to stick with certain guidelines. DSHEA allows four categories of structure/function claims on dietary supplements:

- Statements of a benefit related to a classical nutrient deficiency (e.g., vitamin C prevents scurvy)
- Statements that describe the role of a nutrient intended to affect the structure or function of the body (e.g., cranberry supports the health of the urinary tract)

- Statements that describe the mechanism by which the nutrient affects the structure or function of the body (e.g., cranberry prevents the adherence of bacteria to the urinary tract cell wall)
- Statements that describe general well-being from the consumption of a particular dietary ingredient (e.g., ginseng supports a sense of well-being)

Using these guidelines, an acceptable example of a structure/function statement for calcium might be "promotes bone health." It would not be allowed to say that calcium "prevents osteoporosis." In April 1998, the FDA modified their position on the 1994 DSHEA and redefined their definition of disease. The FDA considered menopause, aging, pregnancy, and even balding and graying as diseases. Since dietary supplements cannot be used to treat a disease, words such as menopause could not appear on the label of any supplement. This often made it difficult for a person to know exactly what a given supplement was for, because the label could not come right out and tell you.

The FDA received 235,000 comments from the public about this decision including 213,000 in the form of letters from consumer and trade groups and 22,000 as individual letters from consumers, members of industry, and other interested parties.[7] In response, the FDA held public meetings in July and August of 1999 to gather more information.

The end result was that things changed. On January 6, 2000, the FDA issued its final regulations on structure/function claims for dietary supplements under the DSHEA. Conditions that are associated with normal life stages are no longer considered diseases, and manufacturers can make structure/function claims for products aimed at helping them. It still is confusing. For instance, "relief of occasional constipation" would be allowed but "chronic constipation" would not, because it could be a symptom of a serious disease. Similarly, "improves absentmindedness" is all right because it does not imply Alzheimer's disease, but "improves memory loss" might and would not be allowed. Every supplement manufacturer must keep a file of scientific papers and other material to substantiate that the claims they make are both true and not misleading. In addition, the following disclaimer must appear in boldface type:

> This statement has not been evaluated by the Food and Drug Administration. This product is not intended to diagnose, treat, cure, or prevent any disease.

Many people who read this warning are unaware that the FDA requires that it be there. The manufacturer must notify the FDA no later than 30 days after marketing the dietary supplement that such a statement is being made. According to the *Prevention* magazine survey, two thirds of consumers remember this statement while one third do not. For 31% it makes the consumer more skeptical about the benefits of a product and for 24%, it makes them less likely to purchase it.

UNDERSTANDING LABELS—WHY IS THERE SAND IN MY CAPSULE?

As you might expect, labels must state what is in a particular product. Reading the labels will help you to do comparison shopping, not only for price but also for content. Before you read your next label, it is helpful to know that until recently, only the main ingredients had to be listed. But now all ingredients are listed. This seems both reasonable and good. But it also causes confusion for consumers because most people do not know what usually goes into the majority of tablets and capsules.

For instance, some of the herbs turn into fine powders once they are ground up. If you ran some through your fingers it would feel like baby powder. Manufacturers put tens of pounds of the stuff into a large funnel that eventually passes through smaller and smaller pipes and tubes until a small amount plops into a capsule. If the funnel only has the fine powder and they turn on the machine, powder flies everywhere except into the capsule. It also sticks to the walls of the pipes and tubes as it flows through at rapid speeds and starts to heat up. Unless something is done about this problem it will either gum up the machine or start a fire.

So how do they fix the problem? Easy: they add small amounts of specific inert material to the powder and suddenly everything is humming. These inert materials are called excipients and they go into just about every OTC supplement and prescription medication sold. Two common examples are sand (also called silicon), because it helps the powder flow, and dicalcium phosphate, which helps prevent the powder from sticking. Bad as it sounds, without it and a few other goodies like it there would not be many tablets or capsules for sale. Usually the excipients are listed last on the labels because they are smallest in quantity. An example of a typical label is shown in Figure 9-1.

WHO SELLS HERBS?

Just about everybody. Huge companies to small companies, grocery stores, drugstores, health food stores, Internet shops, and on and on. Until recently, most drug companies were not interested in producing herbal products, because the plants could not be patented. There was no way the drug companies could recover the $300 million to $800 million it takes for them to bring a new drug to market. However, over the last few years there has been a big change. Larger companies are entering the herbal market with their own brands hoping to protect their products by using patented methods of extracting a particular herb from a plant or by using standardized extracts that they

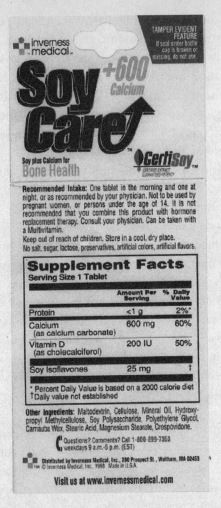

FIGURE 9-1.   Supplement Label Showing All Ingredients
SOURCE: Inverness Medical, Inc., Waltham, Massachusetts.

import from European or American pharmaceutical firms. Here are some examples:

- **Inverness Medical, Inc.:** SoyCare Menopause (soy extract), SoyCare Bone Health (soy extract, calcium, and vitamin D)

- **Warner-Lambert:** Quanterra brands (ginkgo, saw palmetto, alerian, ginger, St. John's wort, and kava kava)
- **Bayer Corporation:** One-a-Day products, Cold Season (echinacea, zinc, and vitamin C), Cholesterol Health (garlic, soy extract, vitamin E, and lecithin), Tension and Mood (St. John's wort and kava kava), Memory (ginkgo and B vitamins), Prostate Health (saw palmetto and zinc), and Menopause Health (black cohosh and soy)
- **Whitehall-Robins Healthcare:** six Centrum Herbal formulas (echinacea, garlic, ginkgo biloba, ginseng, saw palmetto, and St. John's wort)
- **Pharmaton (Boehringer Ingelheim):** Venastat (horse chestnut seed extract to promote better circulation in the legs), Movana (St. John's wort), Ginkgoba and Ginsana (ginseng capsules and chewy squares)
- **Lichtwer Pharma:** Ginkai (ginkgo), Kira (St. John's wort), and Kwai (garlic)
- **Rexall Sundown:** Ginkgo, milk thistle, St. John's wort, and saw palmetto
- **PhytoPharmica:** Remifemin (black cohosh), Remifemin Plus (black cohosh plus St. John's wort)

Hopefully companies will bring improved quality and safety credibility to these products and to the herbal industry. But be prepared to pay for these improvements with a higher price.

LABELS AND DOSAGES

When you read a label on the back of a product there are some things you should consider.

Is the dosage therapeutic? Now that herbals are so popular, the makers of food, candy, drinks, and more, as well as the makers of nutritional supplements, are sprinkling in one herb or another in order to distinguish their product. Make certain that you understand how much of a particular herb you must take to expect a possible benefit. Many of the brands do not put enough in to be therapeutic. When we talk about the major herbs that women are taking I'll point out the proper dosage. For many of the herbs on the market there are no recommended daily amounts. You must either know how much to take by reading the existing studies or know who to ask for this information.

Realize that the dosage listed on the label may not mean the proper dosage is actually in the pill. The *Boston Globe* went around to a number of stores and purchased St. John's wort and then sent samples from each bottle for independent testing. The results were appalling. Some of the products had only a small percentage of what they had written on the label.[8] Realize that quality costs more money (if it sounds too inexpensive to be true, it probably is not a bargain at all), but more money does not guarantee quality.

INDEPENDENT TESTING

Until recently, there was no easy way to know which brands were of high quality. In the past year, an independent laboratory has begun to test categories of supplements and publishes their findings on the Internet at *www.ConsumerLab.com*. Those products that meet quality-testing standards are published on the site. The only problem is that if you do not see your favorite brand, you will not know whether the product failed or simply was not tested.

HERBS AND SAFETY

Although the majority of herbs are safe, and herbs as a group are safer than prescription drugs, the more you know the safer you will be. Why take extra chances? Be sure and tell your doctor or health-care provider if you take any over-the-counter preparations, no matter how safe they may seem. Almost any herb can cause a problem for some people, especially if they are taking other medications or supplements at the same time. Sometimes a vitamin or herb can raise the level of an existing medication and sometimes it can lower the level. Some adverse drug effects and drug interactions are listed below.

TABLE 9-3. DRUG INTERACTIONS WITH SELECTED HERBS AND FOODS

Drug	Herb/Food	Adverse Effect/Interaction
Alprazolam	Kava	Enhances central nervous system activity of alprazolam
Amantadine	Quinine	Increased amantadine, which can cause toxicity with symptoms such as mental confusion
Amoxicillin/Ampicillin	Khat	Delay or decrease absorption of amoxicillin and ampicillin
Astemizole	Grapefruit juice	Increases astemizole activity
Buspirone	Grapefruit juice	Increases buspirone levels
Calcium channel blockers (amlodipine, felodipine, nifedipine, nisoldipine)	Grapefruit juice	Increases levels: amlodipine 15%, felodipine >300%, nifedipine 35%, nisoldipine 400%
Carbamazepine	Grapefruit juice	Increases drug levels 40%
	Quinine	Increases drug levels 37%
Cyclosporin	Grapefruit juice St. John's wort	Increases drug levels and usual side effects
Digoxin	Quinine	Increases levels 75%
	Licorice	Increases levels fourfold
	Hawthorn	increases heart toxicity
	St. John's wort	Decreases levels 25%
Estrogen	Grapefruit juice	Increases levels 37%
Lithium	Herbs with diuretic properties (broom, buchu, dandelion, juniper)	Increases serum levels

(continued)

TABLE 9-3. DRUG INTERACTIONS
WITH SELECTED HERBS AND FOODS *(continued)*

Drug	Herb/Food	Adverse Effect/Interaction
Midazolam	Grapefruit juice	Increases serum levels
Paroxetine and other selective serotonin reuptake inhibitors	St. John's wort	Incoherence, confusion, nausea, weakness, and fatigue; effects occurred 10 days after paroxetine stopped and first dose of St. John's wort begun
Phenelzine	Panax Ginseng (Asian)	Insomnia, tremulousness, tension headaches, irritability, and visual hallucinations
Phenobarbital	Quinine	Increases drug levels 35%
Quinidine	Grapefruit juice	Decreases and delays heart effects
Spironolactone	Licorice	Loss of potassium and muscle weakness
Theophylline	St. John's wort	Increases serum levels 50%
Triazolam	Grapefruit juice	Increases serum levels
Warfarin	Danshen	Increases blood thinning
	Ginkgo biloba, garlic, feverfew, and cayenne	Increases risk of bleeding/bruising
	Licorice	Increases blood-thinning activity
	Alfalfa	Reduces blood-thinning activity
	Vitamin E (>200 IU/day)	Increases blood-thinning activity
	Ginger	Increases blood-thinning activity
	Quinine	Increases blood-thinning activity

POPULAR HERBS FOR MENOPAUSE

Although there is still a lot we do not know about even the most popular herbs, more information is becoming available all the time. This section will focus on the most popular herbs used for menopause and make you aware of the benefits and risks of taking them. Remember, always check with your doctor when you start taking an herb. Most are safe, many are helpful, but all could potentially cause side effects in some people or interact with other medications you might be taking. In particular, be cautious about taking herbs before surgery. Ginkgo, garlic, ginger, ginseng, and feverfew may increase bleeding. Ginseng may affect blood pressure.[9] Other herbs such as St. John's wort, kava kava, and valerian may interact with anesthetics. These potential risks caused the American Society of Anesthesiologists to advise that herbal medicines should not be taken 2 to 3 weeks before elective surgery.

Black Cohosh

BOTANY

Black cohosh is one of the more common herbs used for the hot flashes associated with menopause and one of the more studied herbs. Its Latin name is *Cimicifuga racemosa*, but it has also been called bugbane, squawroot, rattleroot, rattlesnakeroot, and black snakeroot.[10] Black cohosh is a member of the Ranunculaceae (buttercup) family and it grows best at the edges of dense forests, from Ontario to Tennessee and west to Missouri. It also grows in Europe, North Asia, and parts of Arctic Siberia. It is a very hardy perennial and I have it growing in my backyard. Each plant can grow to 6 feet tall and is topped by a long plume of small white flowers that bloom from June to September. The term "black" refers to the dark color of its rhizome or rootstock. Cohosh comes from the Algonquian word for "rough," because that is how the rhizome feels.

HISTORY

Black cohosh has a long history in folk medicine, especially among the Native Americans who boiled the root in water and drank the resulting beverage. It has been used to treat painful periods, the pain of childbirth, upset stomach, and the symptoms of arthritis. A tea of the root has also been recommended for soothing a sore throat. The plant is named for Latin words *cimex* (bug) and *fuga* (repel) because the plant causes insects, especially cygus bugs, to strictly avoid it. For that reason, black cohosh has been used as a bug repellent as well. Around the turn of the last century, an old-time remedy called Lydia Pinkham's Vegetable Compound contained black cohosh along with many other natural ingredients. In the mid-1950s a German company standardized black cohosh into the brand-name product Remifemin that is now sold in the United States. Many other preparations are also available.

CHEMISTRY

There are many reports from Germany on the chemistry of black cohosh in the European literature dating back to the late 1960s. Many substances have been identified in black cohosh, such as the alkaloids N-methylcysteine, tannins, and terpenoids (acetin, 12-acetylactein, and cimigoside). Black cohosh also contains acetic, butyric, formic, isoferulic, oleic, palmitic, and salicylic acids, recemosin.[11] Other substances in black cohosh include phytosterols, acteina (a resinous mixture), and volatile oil.[12] About 15% to 20% of the root is made of an amorphous resinous substance called cimicifugin. The constituents of black cohosh that give it its value are triterpenoid glycosides, specifically the xylosides actein and cimifugoside. The effectiveness of black cohosh is based on the total amount of triterpenoid glycosides.[13] But as you can see, there are a lot of other substances within black cohosh, and, for the most part, their specific roles are not clear.[14]

PHARMACOLOGY

There are a number of studies that show how black cohosh works. It appears to act like estrogen in grown mice because black cohosh can cause their uterine weight to increase as well as cause an increased circulation of their genitals. Immature mice given black cohosh develop a 48% increased weight in their ovaries compared to untreated mice.[15] An encouraging laboratory study showed that an extract of cimicifuga slowed down growth in one cell line of breast cancer cells.[16] Other animal studies showed that black cohosh could lower blood pressure, work as an anti-inflammatory agent, and even lower blood sugar.[17]

CLINICAL STUDIES

Black cohosh has been used to treat premenstrual problems, painful periods, and symptoms of menopause since the 1940s.[18] By 1962, at least 14 clinical studies or reports involving over 1,500 patients using black cohosh extract had appeared. Although the studies were not performed as stringently as we would expect today, they did show the herb helped relieve hot flashes and improve some of the mood swings in menopause. Many of those studies used dosages of 20 to 30 drops 1 to 3 times each day.[19] Human studies in the 1980s showed that black cohosh could help menopausal symptoms and was safe. If you use a black cohosh tablet, results are best when the tablet is swallowed unchewed with liquid rather than sucked. A typical dosage is 20 milligrams (mg) twice daily (standardized to 2.5% triterpene glycosides) or you can take 2 to 4 milliliters (ml) of the tincture form of the herb 3 times a day. Alternatively, make a tea by placing 1 teaspoon of the dried root in a cup of water and bring to a boil, then simmer gently for 10 minutes. Some of the major studies are listed in Table 9-4.

SAFETY AND TOXICITY

Too much black cohosh can cause dizziness, nausea, severe headaches, stiffness, and trembling limbs. Occasional stomach pains and intestinal discomfort may also happen, and a slower

TABLE 9-4. CLINICAL STUDIES OF BLACK COHOSH

Author/Year	Number of Women Studied	Dose	Outcome
Stolze, 1982[20]	704	40 drops Remifemin twice daily 3 months	>4 weeks, 80% reported improved symptoms, 7% had stomach complaints
Daiber, 1983[21] Voberg, 1984[22] Warnecke, 1985[23]	36 50 60	40 drops Remifemin twice daily 6–8 weeks 40 drops Remifemin twice daily 3 months Group 1: 40 drops Remifemin twice daily Group 2: Estrogen 0.625 mg daily Group 3: Diazepam, 2 mg daily All 3 groups comparatively good	>4 weeks some improvement Improved mood, less weariness Estrogen and Remifemin both thickened the wall of the vagina
Stoll, 1987[24]	80	Group 1: 2 tabs black cohosh 40 mg (2 tabs twice daily) Group 2: Estrogen 0.625 mg daily Group 3: Placebo	>12 weeks, improved symptoms in black cohosh even more than estrogen, none seen in placebo
Petho, 1987[25]	50	2 tabs black cohosh 40 mg (2 tabs twice daily), estrogen injections also given if symptoms continued	82% found black cohosh good or very good, 58% not need to continue estrogen after coming off it (42% did need at least some estrogen continued)
Lehmann-Willenbrock and Riedel, 1988[26]	60	Group 1: 2 tabs black cohosh 40 mg (2 tabs twice daily) Group 2: Estriol, 1 mg daily Group 3: conjugated estrogen 1.25 mg daily Group 4: Estrogen/Progesterone combined	Improvements of symptoms in all four groups
Duker et al, 1991[27]	110	Group 1: Remifemin tablets, 8 mg daily Group 2: Placebo	Remifemin lowered LH levels but did not affect FSH or prolactin levels

NOTE: LH = luteinizing hormone; FSH = follicle-stimulating hormone.

pulse and perspiration have also been reported.[28] Although one report has shown that black cohosh does not increase breast cancer cell growth in a petri dish,[29] it is far too early to be certain that it is safe to take for women who have had breast cancer. Large dosages of the plant may cause miscarriages. It should not be taken in pregnancy or if breast-feeding. Germany's Commission E, which is similar to our Food and Drug Administration, cautions that the drug should not be taken for more than 6 months without women being seen by their physician, which is also the practice with HRT in Germany. However, the Commission E does approve black cohosh for premenstrual syndrome, menstrual pain, and symptoms associated with menopause.

OTHER ALTERNATIVE TREATMENTS FOR HOT FLASHES

Although there is a fair amount of information about black cohosh for the treatment of hot flashes, there is far less scientific information about a variety of other alternatives commonly used to treat this symptom. This is what you need to know about the ones most commonly used:

Flaxseed

Like many foods with enduring quality, flaxseeds have been consumed for thousands of years. They remain a staple part of the diet in Asia, Scandinavia, and Africa. Flaxseeds look a lot like sesame seeds, except they are dark brown and have a pleasant nutty taste. In ancient times, they were known as linseed and the plant's fibers were woven into linen, paper, and rope. The Egyptians used linen to make the cloth for wrapping mummies.

Flaxseeds contain about 18% protein, and they are a rich source of calcium, potassium, and B vitamins. They are also a source of boron, a micronutrient that is being considered as increasingly important in conditions such as arthritis and which may enhance the levels of the body's own estrogen.

Flaxseeds are a rich source of the phytoestrogens known as lignans, and the major ones are matairesinol and secoisolariciresinol. These in turn are converted into enterolactone and enterodiol respectively by intestinal bacteria. For a more complete discussion of the estrogen effects of flax, you might want to read a review article.[30] Many women state that flaxseed has been helpful in reducing their hot flashes, but there is very little scientific data to support their reports.[31] To help with hot flashes, try 1 to 2 tablespoons of flaxseed oil daily, grind up flaxseeds and spread them on your salad or add them to your cereal, or consider some of the new flax and soy products distributed by Zoe Foods (*www.zoefoods.com*) and others that make cereals and bars. I particularly like the idea of adding soy and flax for hot flashes to merge the benefits of both.

Flaxseeds are also high in soluble fiber. In fact, soaking flaxseeds overnight in water turns them into a gelatinous mass that makes a gentle fiber and a great cooking ingredient. You can also grind up the seeds to make flaxseed cereals, crusts, and snack bars. Flaxseeds can also be found as powders, which is more of a laxative than a cooking ingredient, and as flax oil, which usually does not have many lignans because they stay behind with the residue of the seeds. Flax oil is a good source of omega-3 fatty acids. Be sure to buy only fresh, refrigerated flax oil in opaque bottles that have an expiration date. Flax oil, when it is fresh, has a nutty taste. When it is old it tastes bitter, even a bit like fish oil. Throw it out and buy a new bottle.

Chasteberry

Chasteberry is the dried, ripe fruit of the chaste tree, *Vitex agnus-castus*. It has been used since antiquity and is mentioned in the early works of Hippocrates, Dioscorides, and Theophrastus around the fourth century B.C. Hippocrates recommended the plant for injuries, inflammation, and swelling of the spleen, and suggested using the leaves in wine to help control hemorrhages and the "passing of afterbirth." The name *agnus castus* comes from the Latin meaning chaste lamb, because it was believed that its seeds taken as a drink had the ability to reduce sexual desire. The English name of chaste tree comes from the belief that taking the plant would suppress the libido of women taking it. This belief led to placing the blossoms of the plant at the clothing of novice monks to supposedly suppress libido.

The fruit of the chasteberry contains about 0.5% volatile essential oils, iridoid glycosides (agnoside and aucubin), and flavonoids. Many British women use it for hot flashes to help balance estrogen and progesterone levels. The only real scientific information on chasteberry are studies showing that taking an extract of the berry could lower the hormone prolactin, the hormone responsible for milk production.[32] Pour 1 cup of boiling water over 1 teaspoon of fresh berries and then steep for 10 minutes to make tea and drink it up to 3 times daily. You can also take 1 ml of the tincture of the herb 3 times a day.

The Commission E recommends chasteberry only for irregularities of the menstrual cycle, premenstrual complaints, and painful breasts. According to that body, menopause is not an indication. There are no published papers on chasteberry and hot flashes. Although there are few studies using this herb, there are no reports of overdose or serious side effects. However, occasional itching and welts have been reported.

Dong Quai

Dong quai is a traditional Chinese herb that has become very popular in the United States as a treatment for a variety of women's health concerns, among them menopause. It is extracted from the

Angelica sinensis root. In China, dong quai is typically prescribed as part of a mixture that includes several other herbs in combination. However, in the United States it is typically sold as a single herb. Some menopausal women do report that dong quai helps relieve hot flashes, but there is little scientific evidence. In 1 study of 71 postmenopausal women, dong quai at a dosage of 4.5 mg daily and a placebo were compared for their ability to reduce the number of hot flashes over a 24-week period of time.[33] According to this study, there were no differences in the number of hot flashes, thickness of the vagina, or a number of other symptoms, including joint pain, insomnia, headaches, or fatigue between the two groups. The investigators did point out that it is possible that formulating dong quai along with four or more other herbs as Chinese practitioners recommend might have made a difference. Until we get more studies, the value of dong quai for relieving hot flashes is still unclear. If you want to try it, a tea can be brewed by placing 1 teaspoon of the dried root in a cup of water and bringing it to a boil, then simmering gently for 10 minutes. You can also use 1 ml of the tincture form of the herb 3 times daily. It may take several weeks to notice any relief in your hot flashes. Be aware that dong quai is a mild laxative and in some women may cause uterine cramps. A rash may also occur if you get too much sun while taking dong quai.

Evening Primrose

The oil of evening primrose (*Oenothera biennis*) is one of the alternative treatments for menopausal symptoms that is often talked about. This plant is a native of North America and is seen along the roads in New England, especially along sandy beaches and the edge of woods, old fields, and ditches. It was brought to Europe in the seventeenth century. It is a biennial that in its first year grows close to the ground, but in its second year shoots up a hairy stem that can reach a height of 3 to 4 feet. It blooms in midsummer and produces large yellow flowers that are followed by downy pods, which contain small seeds.

Native Americans consumed the leaves, roots, and seedpods for food and as prepared extracts for a variety of conditions. Today, evening primrose is used for a number of different conditions including rheumatoid arthritis, eczema, multiple sclerosis, premenstrual syndrome (PMS), cardiovascular disorders, chronic fatigue syndrome, Raynaud's syndrome, weight loss, endometriosis, and diabetes.[34] Herbalists use the flowers and the seeds to press oil that is high in gamma-linolenic acid (GLA) and essential polyunsaturated fatty acids that convert into prostaglandins, hormones necessary for many of the body's functions. The oil of evening primrose also contains linoleic acid plus gamma-linolenic acid, an omega-6 fatty acid that is formed in the human body by the desaturation of linoleic acid. These essential fatty acids (EFAs) are necessary for proper brain and nervous system function. They help maintain the structure and function of cell membranes and promote healthy skin, hair, and nails. They may also reduce blood cholesterol levels.

Although there are a number of good scientific studies using evening primrose oil for eczema and the other conditions, I could find only one study on evening primrose for menopause. Unfortunately it showed no benefit over placebo for hot flashes.[35] That does not mean you should not give it a try if nothing else is working. It is usually well tolerated although mild upset stomach, indigestion, nausea, softening of stools, and headache occasionally have occurred.[36] If you take too much, you can expect loose stools and a stomachache, but no special treatment is required—evening primrose oil is nontoxic. The recommended daily dosage of evening primrose oil is 4 grams (containing around 300 to 360 mg GLA). Most capsules contain about 500 mg and cost 25 cents each, so 4 grams daily amounts to about $2 a day. The only warning is that people with temporal lobe epilepsy or schizophrenia may worsen if they take evening primrose oil along with conventional medications.

Red Clover

Red clover (*Trifolium pratense*) is another plant that contains phytoestrogens—in this case formononetin, biochanin A, daidzein, and genistein. It has also been used for treatment of menopausal symptoms. Two clinical trials from Australia were unable to demonstrate that red clover extract was any better than using a placebo.[37, 38] However, another study using a dose of 40 mg a day did find a significant reduction in hot flashes.[39] There is still too little information to know whether or not red clover will have any effect on the uterine lining or on breast tissue. Because red clover contains coumarins, which have the ability to thin the blood, high dosages may cause this problem as well.

Tablets are available on the market and dosages of 40 mg daily are recommended and are marketed as Promensil. It can also be taken as a tea by placing boiling water over 1 to 3 teaspoons of dried herb and letting steep for 10 minutes 3 times daily or as 1 to 2 ml tincture 3 times daily. Allergic reactions have been reported.[40]

Vitamin E

We have all heard about using vitamin E as an antioxidant, but there are a number of anecdotes that suggest it may be helpful for hot flashes as well. There were some studies using vitamin E in the 1940s and 1950s, but most were poorly designed and did not compare their findings with a placebo group. One study did compare vitamin E with estrogen and a placebo for hot flashes and 10 other symptoms and did not find the vitamin E to be any better than the placebo.[41] However, because the scientists were evaluating 11 different symptoms and not just hot flashes, that conclusion may not be fair. More recently another study using 400 international units (IU) of vitamin E twice daily was compared with a placebo in 125 breast cancer survivors with at least 14 hot flashes a week. The patients taking vitamin E had on average 1 less hot flash per day.[42] At present, the value of vitamin E for hot flashes seems minimal. If you want to try it, doses of up to 1,000 IU daily appear to be safe with little in the way of risk or side effects. If you are also taking aspirin or ginkgo at the same time you are taking higher amounts of vitamin E, be careful. Increased blood thinning can occur, causing internal bleeding and easy bruising.

Ginkgo Biloba

BOTANY

The ginkgo is the oldest living tree species on this planet. It can be traced back more than 200 million years to fossils of the Permian period. The ginkgo is the only survivor of the Ginkgoaceae family. Although it is native to China, it was brought to Europe in 1730 and now grows in temperate climates in many parts of the world. Ginkgo trees grow to nearly 125 feet and have fan-shaped leaves. The species is dioecious; male trees more than 20 years old blossom in the spring. Adult female trees produce a plumlike gray-tan fruit that falls in late autumn. The pulp of these fruits smells foul and can irritate the skin. However, the almond-shaped seed is edible and is sold in Oriental markets. Because the ginkgo tree is highly resistant to insects and parasites, it can live for thousands of years. After the bombing of Hiroshima in 1945, it was the sprout of a ginkgo tree that was the first growth to appear.

HISTORY

Ginkgo has been used in Chinese medicine since 2800 B.C. when Emperor Shen Nung (2839–2698 B.C.) published it as part of the Chinese medicinal text *Pen T'sao Ching*. The emperor, who is considered the first Chinese herbalist, explained that the leaves enhanced cognitive abilities. He, along with other Chinese herbalists, believed that ginkgo leaves helped relieve the symptoms of asthma and bronchial cough while the seeds were an aid to digestion.

CHEMISTRY

Ginkgo contains two groups of active compounds and their subsets:

- Ginkgo flavonoid glycosides (includes three bioflavonoids): quercetin, kaempferol, isorhamnetin
- Terpene lactones: ginkgolides A, B, and C; bilobalide

In Germany and France, extracts of ginkgo are made from dried leaves in a multistep procedure. The monograph published by Germany's Commission E describes the medicinal ginkgo extracts as having 22% to 27% flavonoid glycosides, 5% to 7% terpene lactones, less than 5 parts per million (ppm) of ginkgolic acids, and small amounts of other chemicals. You may come across extracts listed as EGb 761 and LI 1370. These are technical names given to the extracts felt to be suitable for use in drug manufacturing in Germany.[43]

Animal studies have shown that ginkgo "thins the blood" by causing platelets to take longer to stop bleeding.[44] Ginkgolide B helps to prevent blood clots from forming. Ginkgolides also relax smooth muscles, which helps open airways in people with asthmalike symptoms.[45]

PHARMACOLOGY

Ginkgo is one of the better-studied herbs and one of the most popular plant extracts both in Europe and in the United States. Its potential benefits have been evaluated for the treatment of just about every type of ailment from the neck up—cerebral insufficiency, dementia, circulatory disorders, vertigo, tinnitus, and headache, and it has also been looked at as a possible treatment for asthma and as a possible antioxidant, scavenging free radicals. When ginkgo extract was injected into the veins of patients with reduced cerebral blood flow, 70% of patients studied showed an age-related increase. Those between the ages of 30 to 50 years old had a 20% increase compared with a 70% increase in those patients 50 to 70 years old.

Ginkgo has also been tested in Alzheimer's disease.[46] In a study, 327 patients with either Alzheimer's disease or dementia due to other causes took a standardized European extract of ginkgo (120 mg per day of EGb 761) or a placebo for 52 weeks. Those taking ginkgo showed improvement in both their cognitive and their social functioning compared to those taking a placebo. Although a few people who take ginkgo have had bleeding into the brain or eyes,[47, 48] in this particular study, the only two people who had a problem with bleeding were in the placebo group.

Ginkgo has also been studied in 111 patients with intermittent claudication, a condition of blood vessels of the legs causing pain with walking.[49] Those patients treated with the ginkgo extract increased their pain-free walking distance. Other reports have also shown improvement of the pain-free walking distance.[50]

Ginkgo seems to do a lot of good. Be careful if you are also taking aspirin, vitamin E, or anticoagulant (blood-thinning) medication. It may be like doubling the dose and that could cause major problems. The March 1999 issue of *Consumer Reports* pointed out something that may also impact effectiveness. Many brands do not actually give you the amounts listed on the labels, and even the same brand may vary quite a bit. One final word of advice on ginkgo. If you are looking to stave off losing your ability to think, give ginkgo a try. But if you simply want to score higher on your next exam, you will probably get better results by studying harder.

Statins

Statins are not herbs. Not even similar. They are a class of cholesterol-lowering prescription drugs approved by the Food and Drug Administration in 1987. Among those are: Mevacor (lovastatin), Pravachol (pravastatin), Zocor (simvastatin), Lescol (fluvastatin), Lipitor (atorvastatin), and Baycol (cerivastatin). They are an alternative to estrogen if your primary reason for wanting to take a medication is to prevent heart disease and your cholesterol level is elevated. They are the most frequently prescribed medication taken by the 13 million Americans who currently take a cholesterol-lowering medication. According to the November 1, 2000, *Harvard Heart Letter,* you can expect to reduce your total cholesterol levels by 25% and your low-density lipoprotein (LDL) cholesterol levels by 35%. This level of cholesterol-lowering power can lead to a 30% to 40% reduction in nonfatal heart attacks.

Recent information suggests that statins may also lower your risk of suffering a bone fracture due to osteoporosis, the likelihood of developing Alzheimer's disease or other dementias, and possibly even lower your risk of developing colon cancer.[51] There is some indication that statins might lower your risk of heart attack even if your cholesterol level is not elevated.

If you are 50 years of age or over and your LDL cholesterol is over 220 mg/dL, your doctor will probably want to discuss taking a statin (or other cholesterol-lowering drug) with you soon. If you have other risk factors, such as diabetes or being overweight, your doctor might discuss taking a medication for lowering cholesterol at that time.

Overall, statins are safe, but no medication is risk free. Tell your doctor if you develop a fever, or notice any unusual pain, weakness, or tenderness in your muscles. About 1 out of 100 people will develop inflammation of their liver while taking these medications. Your doctor will want to take a blood test to see if your liver enzymes are elevated. If they show that they are elevated, do not worry. Your liver will function normally again once you stop the medication. Co Q-10, an enzyme, in doses of 100 mg twice daily may help prevent these problems. It is wise to limit the amount of alcohol you take while on statins.

Some medications interact with statins in dangerous ways. Be cautious if you are taking the blood thinner warfarin (Coumadin); macrolide antibiotics, such as erythromycin; or the transplant drug cyclosporine. Let your doctor know if you are taking other types of cholesterol-lowering drugs, such as gemfibrozil (Lopid) and niacin (Nicolar), both of which can cause serious interactions.

What if you have an extremely high cholesterol level and statins do not work for you or you find you cannot tolerate them? A study published in the *British Journal of Nutrition* in 1999 showed that in such patients, soybean protein could significantly lower cholesterol, even when only partly replacing animal protein in the diet.[52] Soy is a mighty bean!

TABLE 9-5. SUMMARY OF ALTERNATIVE REMEDIES FOR MENOPAUSE

Herb	Actions	Used For	Dosage	Concerns
Black cohosh (*Cimicifuga racemosa*)—root	Some estrogen activity by attaching to estrogen receptor; lowers luteinizing hormone (LH); may stimulate uterus	Menopausal symptoms (hot flashes, anxiety, and depression) best studied and premenstrual syndrome	All dosages used 2–3 times daily. Tablets 20 mg (standardized to 2.5% triterpene glycosides); extract: 0.3–2.0 ml, 1:10, 60% alcohol	Mild gastrointestinal distress. In high dosages can cause nausea, vomiting, dizziness, low pulse, and perspiration
Chasteberry (*Vitex agnus-castus*)	Increases progesterone by stimulating pituitary gland to make LH. Lowers prolactin, mild sedative, and antispasmodic	PMS symptoms, especially anxiety, depression, moodiness, and sleeplessness. Some menopausal symptoms	Extract—40 drops of liquid, 2 mg twice daily standardized to 0.5% agnoside	Generally considered safe
Echinacea Flower head and leaf better studied than root	Antiviral, immune stimulant, antibacterial, anti-inflammatory	Colds, chronic respiratory and lower urinary tract conditions, wounds, burns, eczema, psoriasis, canker sores, recurrent ear infections	All dosages used 3 times daily. Teas—0.5–1 gram; encapsulated freeze-dried plant—325–600 mg; tincture—(1:5), 2–4 ml; extract—(1:1), 2–4 ml; solid extract to contain 3.5% echinacoside, 150–300 ml	Very few. Caution with autoimmune disease, or medicines that suppress the immune system

(continued)

TABLE 9-5. SUMMARY OF ALTERNATIVE REMEDIES FOR MENOPAUSE (continued)

Herb	Actions	Used For	Dosage	Concerns
Garlic (Allium sativum)—clove	Lower cholesterol, may reduce blood clots by prolonging bleeding and clotting times, fights certain bacteria and viruses, and may reduce risk of stomach cancer	Stomach ailments, respiratory ailments, recurrent colds	Commonly standardized to 4–12 mg allicin daily Available as 400–1 200 mg powder, 2–5 grams fresh dried bulb; oil—0.03–0.12 ml; tincture—2–4 ml (1:5 in 45% alcohol) 3 times daily European preparations standardized to allicin yield	Odorless garlic may be less effective May cause flatulence, heartburn, nausea, vomiting, and unpleasant sensations in your mouth Therapeutic dosages in pregnancy may increase risk of miscarriage
Ginger (Zingiber officinale)—rhizome	Anti-inflammatory, improves circulation, reduces nausea Antispasmodic	Colic, gas, and upset stomach, possibly motion sickness and morning sickness	0.5–2 grams dried rhizome 2–3 times daily, or 1.5–3 ml extract 3 times daily For nausea, 250 mg every 2–3 hours for up to 4 dosages Begin a day before travel to prevent motion sickness	Do not use if you have gallstones Higher dosages may cause miscarriage, but herbalists recommend 1–2 grams dried root or prepared ginger daily for morning sickness Excessive dosages should be discussed with medical provider if you are taking diabetes or heart medication

(continued)

TABLE 9-5. SUMMARY OF ALTERNATIVE REMEDIES FOR MENOPAUSE (continued)

Herb	Actions	Used For	Dosage	Concerns
Ginkgo (Ginkgo biloba)—dried leaf extract; contains 22%–27% flavone glycosides, 5%–7% terpene lactones (ginkgolides A, B, C, and bilobalide), and no more than 5 ppm ginkgolic acids Seeds also used	Reduces blood clot formation, improves brain circulation and oxygen use by brain, improves painful walking due to poor circulation	Memory lapses, difficulty concentrating, emotional depression, dizziness, tinnitus, and headache Inhaling decoction of leaves used to treat asthma; seeds used for cough and congestion	Leaf extract: 80–240 mg daily Solid extract: 40 mg 3 times daily Fluid extract: (1:1) 0.5 ml three times daily	Generally considered safe Gastrointestinal upset and headache reported Seed can cause food poisoning Extracts taken with blood thinners, vitamin E, or aspirin may cause bleeding
Ginseng (Panax ginseng)—root White ginseng is the peeled, sun-dried root; red ginseng is unpeeled, steamed, and dried. Root contains at least 1.5% ginsenosides, calculated as ginsenoside Rg 1	Lowers blood sugar, stimulant, anti-inflammatory, may improve mental function	Tonic for invigorating and fortifying when feeling fatigue or debility, and for reduced ability to work and concentrate	For young and healthy: 0.5–1.0 gram of root daily as 2 divided dosages Usually used for 15–20 days with a 2-week root-free period Best taken in morning 2 hours before a meal, and in the evening at least 2 hours after a meal For old and sick: 0.4–0.8 gram root daily Break not needed	Generally safe Use with caution for cardiac patients or patients with diabetes, and those using monoamine oxidase (MAO) inhibitor medications

(continued)

TABLE 9-5. SUMMARY OF ALTERNATIVE REMEDIES FOR MENOPAUSE (continued)

Herb	Actions	Used For	Dosage	Concerns
Ginseng, Siberian (Eleutherococcus senticosus)—dried root and rhizome	Stimulates immune system, raises blood pressure, involved in digestive and glucose regulation	Chronic inflammation, chronic fatigue syndrome, fibromyalgia, and chemotherapy Used to revive strength and energy	2–3 grams dried and powdered root and rhizome daily; solid extracts standardized at 300–400 mg eleutherosides B and E daily, or 8–10 ml 2–3 times daily Usually taken for 6–8 weeks with 1 week off and another 6–8 week course	Use with caution when taking stimulants, antipsychotics, heart or blood pressure medications Avoid if pregnant or breastfeeding At higher dosages, insomnia, anxiety, irritability, and palpitations occur
Licorice root (Liquiritiae radix)—unpeeled, dried roots and stolons of Glycyrrhiza glabra	Increases healing of ulcers; helps break up respiratory secretions	Inflammation of the mucous membranes of the upper respiratory tract and stomach or duodenal ulcers	5–15 grams of root, equivalent to 200–600 mg of glycyrrhizin	Can increase loss of potassium, therefore use with caution with diuretics and digitalis Do not use more than 4–6 weeks without medical advice

(continued)

TABLE 9-5. SUMMARY OF ALTERNATIVE REMEDIES FOR MENOPAUSE (continued)

Herb	Actions	Used For	Dosage	Concerns
Soy (isoflavones are the major active ingredient)	Natural plant estrogen (phytoestrogen), inhibits growth of some cancer cells, slows down loss of calcium from bones, lowers cholesterol, improves elasticity of arteries, reduces hot flashes	Menopausal symptoms, helps prevent osteoporosis, promotes heart health, may reduce risk of breast, prostate, and colon cancer	Soymilk—8 ounces daily; tofu or soy nuts—half cup daily; soy protein—40–50 grams (usually two scoops) daily; capsules/tablets—25 mg isoflavones twice daily maintain blood levels throughout the day	Generally considered safe May cause flatulence
St. John's wort (Hypericum perforatum)—above ground parts	Antibiotic, reduces inflammation in topical preparations, sedative and tranquilizing effect on brain	Treatment of mild depression Used externally to treat wounds and burns	Tablets 600–900 mg daily in divided dosages standardized to 0.2% hypericin or 2–4 grams of total herb	May cause rash in sunlight May interact with antidepressant medications Medical professional should treat severe depression

TABLE 9-6. CLASSES OF CHOLESTEROL-LOWERING DRUGS

Drug Class	Metabolic Effects	Concerns
Niacin (nicotinic acid)	Lowers LDL-C 10% to 25%, lowers TG 20% to 30%, raises HDL-C 10% to 35%	Can raise blood glucose and uric acid levels, can be toxic to liver, cause stomach ulcers, and frequently causes skin flushing, itching, nausea, and abdominal discomfort. Only 50% to 60% can tolerate for long periods of time
Bile acid sequestrants (cholestyramine, colestipol)	Lowers LDL-C 10% to 30% by binding bile acids in the intestines	May raise TG, frequent intestinal problems cause it to often be stopped; many drug interactions; may lower absorption of folic acid and fat-soluble vitamins D, A, K, and E
HMG-CoA reductase inhibitors (statins)	Primarily lowers LDL-C 15% to 40% by interfering with cholesterol synthesis in the liver	Can inflame the liver, so check liver enzymes; muscle aches and fatigue in a small number of patients
Fibric acid derivatives (gemfibrozil, fenofibrate)	Primarily lowers TG 30% to 55%, raises HDL-C 15% to 25% by stimulating the enzyme lipoprotein lipase	Fenofibrate may lower total cholesterol and LDL-C 20% to 25%; both raise LDL-C but transform it into a less artery-hardening form. Gemfibrozil may raise LDL-C 10% to 15%; many intestinal symptoms, possible gallstones, and severe possible interactions with other drugs; can raise homocysteine levels independent of vitamin concentrations

NOTE: LDL-C = low-density lipoprotein cholesterol; HDL-C = high-density lipoprotein cholesterol; TG = triglycerides; HMG-CoA = coenzyme A

chapter 10

INCORPORATING SOY INTO YOUR LIFE

No illness which can be treated by diet should be treated by any other means.

Moses Maimonides, A.D. 1200

Never in the history of nutrition research has the evidence been more clear and consistent. A high-carbohydrate, low-calorie, plant-based diet is the best for long term health.

Bradley J. and D. Craig Wilcox, authors of The Okinawa Program, *quoted in the* Boston Globe, May 22, 2001

Okinawa, the chain of islands near Japan, has an enviable new position in the world—it is the home of the world's longest-living people with a higher percentage of 100-year-olds than anyplace else. Okinawa's centenarian rate is 3 to 6 times higher than the United States'. Why? According to Richard Saltus in a front-page health and science article in the *Boston Globe* (May 22, 2001): "In stark contrast to American habits, Okinawans eat a vegetable-based diet low in both calories and fats, and rich in soy foods, and they exercise regularly."

It is ironic that as Okinawans are beginning to go astray with the invasion of fast-food chains and other Western lifestyle fads, Americans are embracing soy. Without question, the new millen-

TABLE 10-1. LIFE EXPECTANCY IN YEARS

Rank	Country	Life Expectancy
1	Japan	74.5
2	Australia	73.2
3	France	73.1
4	Sweden	73.0
5	Spain	72.8
24	United States	70.0

NOTE: Life expectancy is for a baby born in 1999, from a World Health Organization study of 191 countries.
SOURCE: Modified from *Boston Globe*, May 22, 2001.

TABLE 10-2. FREQUENCY OF CENTENARIANS

Location	100-Year-Olds per 10,000
Okinawa	34
Nova Scotia	20
New England	10
England/Wales	8

SOURCE: World Health Organization, New England Centenarian Study, Max Planck Institute. Compiled by the *Boston Globe*, May 22, 2001.

nium has seen soy go from zero to hero. Whether in the form of pea-size soybeans, chewy cubes of tofu, or creamy glasses of soymilk, the soy foods market has skyrocketed. Peter Golbitz, president of Soyatech, Inc., a major manufacturer of soy foods in Bar Harbor, Maine, told the *Boston Globe* his company had just completed a market study that found that overall soy food sales in 1998 were $1.75 billion. He said he expected it to rise to $2.6 billion in the year 2000.

Consumption of soy nutritional supplements is also on the rise. According to Information Resources, Inc. (IRI), the total soy supplement category has gone from $842,000 for all of 1997 to over $40.2 million for the 52-week period ending February 4, 2001. These data underestimate soy nutritional supplement consumption because they include only food, drug, and mass merchandising outlets. They omit gas stations, convenience stores, wholesale clubs (such as BJ's or Costco), discount stores, health food stores, and direct and on-line purchases. Supermarket sales of soy also soared between 1998 and 1999. Tofu sales increased 19% to $46 million, soymilk sales increased 85% to $77.4 million, and soy energy bars increased 93% to $81.6 million. In 2000, soymilk sales alone increased to $420 million.[1]

An annual survey conducted by the United Soybean Board (USB) and reported in October 2000, found that Americans' consumption of soy continues to rise along with their recognition of soy's health benefits. Of American consumers, 76% consider soy products to be healthful, 39% are aware of soy's specific health benefits, and 27% are altering their eating habits to include soy products one or more times each week. These percentages include men and women, young and old; so the numbers of menopausal women consuming soy are likely to be much higher than reported.

The November 1999 HRS (*Health Supplement Retailer*) stated, "Soy—it appears—has gone mainstream." Judy Foreman summed it up in a February 15, 2000, front-page health and science *Boston Globe* article, "Americans have fallen in love with the humble soybean."

OLD HABITS DIE HARD

Though American appreciation of the many health benefits of soy is growing, there are those who still think it is not possible to live without meat. For example, hundreds of people gathered outside a butcher shop in Panzano in Chianti, Italy, and bid up to $5,000 for a special cut of T-bone weighing four pounds as the last of an outlawed meat supply went from the butcher block to the auction block.[2] Neither mad cow disease nor foot and mouth disease nor the fact that many of the world's major chronic diseases could be prevented or reduced in frequency by "steering" clear of beef and other animal proteins and consuming a primarily vegetarian diet deterred them. Old habits die hard.

UNDERSTANDING SOY FOODS

Soy is a tremendous source of protein, minerals, vitamins, and other health benefits. Many people are unfamiliar with the various forms of soy available and soy's tremendous nutritional value.

Soy is a truly versatile food. There are many ways to prepare it, and many ways to incorporate it into your diet. If you think soy is an acquired taste that may not be for you, read on.

Soy Sprouts

Soybeans can be sprouted. It takes about 5 to 10 days for beans to sprout. Soy sprouts look a lot like mung bean sprouts, and they are an excellent source of magnesium, folic acid, and, unlike almost every other form of soy, vitamin C. Soy sprouts can be added fresh to salads or cooked fast at low heat. Unlike some soybean products, soy sprouts are low in sodium.

Soybeans and Soy Foods Made Directly from Them

SOYBEANS

Soybeans eaten whole are the simplest form of soy food. They grow in fuzzy green pods with two to three beans in each pod on bushy plants 2 to 3 feet tall. Soybeans come in a variety of colors, depending on when they are harvested. If they are freshly harvested when they are still slightly immature, soybeans are green in color and look like Chinese snow peas. You may see these called edamame. Late in the growing season, when they are fully mature, the green soybeans begin to dry and turn yellow, black, or brown. At this stage they look like black-eyed peas without the black eye.

You can eat fresh soybeans as a snack or as an appetizer by boiling or steaming them in the pod for 10 to 15 minutes. Chill them, and serve them fanned out on a platter, lightly salted. Be sure to peel off the pods before eating them. You can also prepare fresh soybeans by removing them from their pods and boiling them in water for 15 to 20 minutes until they are tender. Not all stores carry fresh soybeans, so if you garden, try growing them at home and harvesting your own supply of soybeans each summer. You can also find whole soybeans that have been harvested, dried, and sold in bags or soybeans that are precooked and canned.

Canned soybeans are ready to use and can be added to chilies, stews, and soups right out of the can. Using the liquid in

TABLE 10-3. EDAMAME: NUTRITIONAL FACTS IN ½ CUP (75 GRAMS)

Calories	90
Total fat	5 grams
Saturated fat	1 gram
Cholesterol	0 mg
Sodium	0 mg
Carbohydrates	3 grams
Dietary fiber	8 grams
Sugar	2 grams
Protein	9 grams
Vitamin C	4%
Calcium	4%

SOURCE: Edamame By Kiyoshi, 398 Harvard Street, Brookline, MA 02446.

the can will save some of the B vitamins that might be lost from the canning process. Dried soybeans, like most other legumes, have to be soaked overnight to rehydrate them. It usually takes about 3 cups of water for each cup of soybeans. In the morning, drain off the water, cover them again with fresh water, and simmer the beans over low heat for 3 hours. Now they are ready to use. Although they may be soft enough to crush with your tongue on the roof of your mouth, do not be surprised if the soybeans are a little chewier than other beans. If your recipe calls for adding a tomato product, add it when the dish is nearly done. Tomatoes tend to toughen the outer layer of the bean, which causes them to take longer to soften.[3] Eat soybeans within a few days once they are cooked.

Roasted soy nuts are high-protein alternatives to peanuts, and have become a popular snack food. They are available in most grocery stores. You can make them yourself: Cover the soybeans with water and soak them for about 3 hours; drain them and spread them out on an oiled cookie sheet. Roast them in a 350° Fahrenheit oven until browned. Salt to taste. If you store them in an airtight container, they should keep for a month at room temperature.

SOY FLOUR

Soy flour is made by grinding up whole dry soybeans. It is dense and moist and cannot be used by itself. But it can replace up to 20% of the weight of all-purpose flour in almost any recipe. Because soy flour is gluten-free, adding more than 20% to bread dough will prevent the bread from rising. Full-fat flour is made from whole soybeans, so it contains all the oil, protein, and dietary fiber you find in the whole bean. According to Ruth Winter in her book *Super Soy: The Miracle Bean*,[4] soy flour is a good choice for doughnut mixes, pancakes, and piecrusts. It adds protein and improves the crust color and shelf life of baked goods.

Oil can be removed from soybeans during processing to make a low-fat or defatted flour. *The Joy of Cooking*[5] suggests that because of its fat content, soy flour can be creamed with the shortening or blended with the liquids rather than mixed with the dry ingredients. It usually comes in 2-pound units. Unlike all-purpose flour, keep your soy flour (full-fat and low-fat) refrigerated or it will go rancid. You can also use soy flour as a substitute for eggs in recipes by adding 1 tablespoon of soy flour and 2 tablespoons of water for each egg called for.

SOY POWDER

Soy powder is very much the same as soy flour, with the exception that the soybeans are cooked before they are ground. The result is a powder that is finer than flour with a reduced beany taste. It can be used to make soymilk or added as powdered milk to coffee. Soy powder can also be added to recipes.

SOY PROTEIN ISOLATES

Soy protein isolates are made by a chemical process that removes most of the protein from defatted soy flour, which results in a textured product that has 90% of the protein with very little moisture. The processing removes the fiber and carbohydrates, but it is an excellent source of protein that can be used to add texture to a variety of soy-based dairy foods, such as cheese, nondairy frozen desserts, and coffee lighteners. Soy protein isolate is also a major component of such varied products as: soy hotdogs, soy ice cream, soy baby food, and soy meat analogues.

TEXTURED VEGETABLE PROTEIN

Textured vegetable protein (TVP) is a modern Western invention made by compressing defatted soy flour until its protein fiber changes in structure. It is a very coarse substance that when rehydrated, has a texture similar to ground beef. Add a little chicken or beef flavoring and you have a stew. You can buy it in bulk or in 1-pound bags. It takes just under a cup of boiling water to rehydrate smaller granules of TVP, but larger chunks must be simmered for several minutes. Most packages provide these instructions. Look for it as a major ingredient in meat substitutes such as sausages or vegetable burgers. When you are cooking, you can add it to hamburger as a meat extender, or use it by itself for tacos or chili. You can use up to 20% of the weight of the recipe, and your taste buds will never know the difference. Your cholesterol levels will benefit—you will be getting 20% less animal fat than the meat version of the same dish.

SOY GRITS

Soy grits are another product that comes from the whole bean. They taste like soybeans and retain 55% to 65% of the protein by weight and most of soy's beneficial contents. They are made by lightly toasting and hulling the soybeans, then either cracking or grinding them into small pieces. Soy grits contain fat, and they can become rancid if not refrigerated. You can use soy grits either as a breakfast cereal by stirring 1 part grits into 3 parts boiling water, cover, and lower the heat. Simmer the grits until all the water is absorbed. This takes about 45 minutes and you do not have to presoak them. Soy grits are a bit chewy, so they are a natural extender for hamburger and a great way to add texture to chili, stews, and spaghetti sauce.

OKARA

Okara is the pulp and hulls that remain after the soymilk is strained. The name means literally "honorable hull." It is very high in fiber and protein. Okara is often described as having a coconut-like texture. It is frequently used in granola bars, muffins, and cookies. It can also be found in vegetarian burgers. Keep your okara refrigerated and use it within a few days.

Soymilk and Products Made from Soymilk

SOYMILK

Soymilk is an ancient drink, developed by the Chinese Buddhist monks who brought it to Japan. It has been a staple beverage throughout Asia ever since, made fresh daily and sold much as we buy cows' milk in the United States. Soymilk has been available in the United States since the 1920s when John Harvey Kellogg of breakfast cereal fame first produced it.

Soymilk is made by soaking, cooking, and pureeing whole soybeans, and then pressing out the milky liquid. It usually comes in airtight, quart-size rectangular cartons with a shelf life of up to 6 months even at room temperature, although some brands come in a glass bottle and require refrigeration. Soymilk powder is also available and must have water added to it. Soymilk comes in a variety of flavors including plain, vanilla, chocolate, carob, and almond. It can be purchased in whole, low-fat, or nonfat versions. Once the carton is opened, it must be refrigerated and used up within a week.

Soymilk has a slightly nutty flavor and can be used for anything you use milk for. I use it on my dry cereal and instead of milk to make cream of wheat and oatmeal cereals. But you can also use it to make sauces, puddings, custards, mousse, or almost anything else you might use cows' milk for. Whole and low-fat soymilk creates a firmer consistency than nonfat. Soymilk is a rich source of iron, phosphorus, thiamin, copper, potassium, and magnesium as well as vegetable protein. If you feel adventuresome, machines to make soymilk are available for home use for about $200. You can find them at Asian food stores and on the Internet.

YUBA

Yuba is the skin that forms on soymilk when it is heated. It is not usually available in the United States, but it can be found widely in China and in gourmet shops in Japan, where it is considered a delicacy. Yuba is 52.4% protein and is commonly added to soups and stews. It can also be pressed into molds and made into imitation meat. Once yuba dries, it becomes brittle and can be deep-fried and made into a chip, or it can be soaked in water to soften, and used to wrap rice or vegetables.[6]

SOY CHEESE

Soymilk can be made into cheeses just as cows' milk can. It is low in fat and cholesterol, and lactose-free. If it is held together with calcium caseinate, that means it contains dairy. If isolated

TABLE 10-4. NUTRITION FACTS—SOYMILK

Serving size	8 fluid ounces	Iron	8%
Total fat	5 grams	Riboflavin (B_2)	4%
Saturated fat	0.5 gram	Niacin (B_3)	4%
Cholesterol	0	Folate	10%
Sodium	105 mg	Magnesium	15%
Potassium	440 mg	Copper	15%
Total carbohydrates	13 grams	Phosphorus	15%
Sugars	7 grams	Zinc	6%
Protein	10 grams	Pyridoxine (B_6)	8%
Calcium	8% daily value	Pantothenic acid (B_5)	6%
Thiamin (B_1)	10%		

SOURCE: Eden Soy Original. Product label.

soy protein is used it is dairy-free. Like soymilk it can be purchased as full-fat, low-fat, or fat-free, as mozzarella, jack, and cheddar. Some of the common brands available in health food stores and supermarkets are Soya-Kaas, Soymage, and Soy-Sation. There is even soy Parmesan and soy cream cheese (under the brand names Tofutti and Soya-Kaas). Higher temperatures cause soy cream cheese to separate, so try cooking with lower temperatures than usually called for.[7]

SOY SOUR CREAM

Soy sour cream uses the same technique as dairy sour cream—a souring agent is added to soymilk. The difference is that soy sour cream contains no cholesterol or lactose and does have about 1 gram of soy protein per serving. Use it exactly as you would dairy sour cream, either as a topping, a spread, or as part of a recipe.

SOY YOGURT

Soy yogurt is another example of a dairy product made from soymilk. Like its dairy counterpart, live bacteria cultures are added to soymilk. A 1-cup serving contains 12 grams of soy protein, no lactose, and no cholesterol. It can be purchased plain or with fruits added and as whole or low fat. Soy yogurt has a similar consistency to dairy yogurt, so you can use it interchangeably for a snack and as an ingredient in sauces, milk shakes, desserts, etc.

TOFU

Tofu is probably one of the most familiar forms of soy. It is also known as bean curd and dou fu-tofu. The Chinese called tofu "meat without bones" or "meat of the fields" because it is such a rich source of protein and minerals. They consume 3 to 4 ounces of it daily. In Japan, tofu has been referred to as o-tofu to bestow it the title of honorable. In addition to its nutrition content, tofu is inexpensive and easily digestible for babies, adults, and the elderly.

Tofu is curdled soymilk. After the curdling agent is added to soymilk it separates into curds and whey. Tofu is the soybean curds that are then compressed into white, spongy cubes seen in most health food stores and supermarkets. The most commonly used curdling agents are salts and which one is used changes the mineral content of the tofu. For instance, nigari, which is a natural sea salt, is the traditional choice. But calcium salts are also commonly used today and tofu made that way is an even richer source of calcium. Tofu comes in several forms. All must be kept refrigerated except the dried variety. For best results, keep any unused portion submerged in water and change the water daily:

- Firm—pressed to remove most of the moisture
- Regular—softer and somewhat more delicate
- Soft—slightly sweeter and softer because it contains slightly more water. Often used for desserts
- Silken—also sweeter and somewhat custardlike
- Smoked—precooked then smoked until brown. Flavorful and firm with cheeselike texture
- Dried—freeze-dried and stored at room temperature. Prepared by boiling in water until it gains a chewy texture. Often found in camping stores
- Age (pronounced AH-gay)—deep-fried cubes of tofu that are hollow inside. Sometimes called tofu pouches

In addition to its nutritional content, tofu is a superb form of soy to cook with because it is bland with no bean flavor. But because it is porous, it is like a flavor sponge—it soaks up the flavor of whatever is cooked with it. Crumble a block of firm tofu in your hand and add it to hamburger and it tastes like hamburger. I like to cut it into cubes and add it to soup or stir-fry it with my favorite seasonings and vegetables. The softer forms of soy are also sweeter and make a great choice for combining with your favorite fruits and whipping them up in the blender. They also make great puddings and cream pies because they take up the taste of the chocolate or whatever flavor you add.

Look for tofu in water-filled containers in the produce section of your supermarket or in aseptically sealed cartons that can be kept on a pantry shelf if unopened. If the slightly sweet smell of your fresh tofu turns slightly sour, you can still use it by boiling it in water for 5 to 10 minutes. In many Asian markets you can buy it in bulk but beware of open containers—they can carry bacterial contamination. If you do not intend to eat it all within a few days, drain out the water, squeeze out any excess water, and put it in the freezer in a well-sealed container. It can be kept there for months but expect the color to darken slightly and the texture to become a little chewier.

Fermented Forms of Soy

TEMPEH

Tempeh (pronounced TEM-pay) is made from whole soybeans. They are cooked with a mold, rhizopus, from the hibiscus plant at a warm temperature for 18 to 24 hours. In Indonesia where tempeh was believed to originate, people make it by placing a

TABLE 10-5. NUTRITION FACTS—FIRM TOFU

Serving size	3 ounces	Total carbohydrates	2 grams
Calories	70	Dietary fiber	<1 gram
Total fat	3.5 grams	Sugars	0
Saturated fat	0.5 gram	Protein	7 grams
Polyunsaturated fat	2.0 grams	Calcium	10%
Monounsaturated fat	1 gram	Iron	14%
Cholesterol	0	Sodium	0

SOURCE: Nasoya firm tofu, a product of Vitasoy, San Francisco, California.

piece of tempeh from a previous batch, called a starter, with the cooked soybeans to begin the fermentation process. At the end of the process, the tempeh emerges as a chunky bean cake covered with an edible white mold.

Tempeh has a strong, distinctive taste with a chewy consistency that makes it a great meat substitute. You can marinate it and barbecue or grill it, steam it, or prepare it as you would tuna fish by grating it up and mixing it with mayonnaise, celery, and onions. A 3-ounce serving has about 150 calories, 16 grams of protein, and 6 grams of fiber. It you notice small gray or black flecks in your tempeh, it just means that it is naturally fermented. The fermentation process actually increases the protein and vitamin B content of tempeh. Tempeh is higher in fiber and lower in fat than either tofu or soymilk. Keep it refrigerated for up to a week or frozen for up to several months.

NATTO

Natto is another fermented soy food made from cooked whole soybeans. It is made by mixing in a bacteria culture with the soybeans and allowing them to ferment in plastic bags. In Japan it is used as a spread, at breakfast or dinnertime, or with shoyu (traditional soy sauce) and mustard. Natto is high in protein content and rich in fiber but lower in sodium than either miso or soy sauce. It's also a good source of iron, minerals, and B vitamins. If you are taking a class of antidepressants called monoamine oxidase (MAO) inhibitors, be careful eating natto. It contains the amino acid tyramine, which can dangerously elevate your blood pressure.

MISO

Miso is made with soybeans alone (called hacho) or soybeans combined with a grain such as barley (called mugi) or rice (called kome) together with salt and a mold culture for up to 3 years in a cedar vat to ferment. It comes in both a smooth and a chunky variety. Since miso is made from a variety of combinations, it may vary greatly in flavor. You might have seen it in miso soup when you eat at Japanese restaurants. It has a wonderfully distinct taste but it is salty. A tablespoon of miso has 680 milligrams (mg) of sodium. Table salt has 6,589 mg of sodium. Miso is a great source of protein (12% to 21%), comparable to eggs (13%) or even chicken (20%). Like natto, it contains the amino acid tyramine that can increase your blood pressure if you are taking a class of antidepressants known as MAO inhibitors.

SOY SAUCE

Everyone who has gone out for Chinese food sees soy sauce either on the table or in the bag when you bring take-out home. The soy sauce we know in America is different from the traditional soy sauce in Asia, which is known as shoyu. Shoyu is made by adding a mold to cooked soybeans and a grain, then fermenting the mixture in a salty brine for 1 to 1½ years.[8] The bottles of soy sauce Americans buy at the supermarket are really defatted soybean meal and wheat mixed with chemicals, corn syrup, and food coloring. Shoyu is sometimes called tamari, but that name is also used for the liquid that is left over when miso is made.

SOY-BASED FOODS

If you are not in the mood to spend time in the kitchen preparing a soy-based meal, there are plenty of soy-based foods already prepared and available in your supermarket, health food store, or from mail-order catalogs. There is soy margarine made primarily or entirely from soy oil, soy mayonnaise made from soybean oil, and "eggs," which is tofu and soybean oil extracted from whole soybeans. None of these contain saturated fat, but they also don't contain any soy protein and usually very small amounts of isoflavones, if any. There is also an increasing variety of meatless products made from soy protein that taste a lot like chicken, beef, tuna, and more. Tofu hot dogs, cheeses, and ice cream are growing in popularity. Keep your eyes out for them at most health food stores and many supermarkets. They are also available over the Internet from places such as Dixie Diner (*www.dixiediner.com*), POB 1969, Tomball, TX 77377, 800-233-3668. It is getting easier and tastier all the time to add soy into your life.

SOY SUPPLEMENTS VERSUS SOY FOOD

In recent years, the interest in nutritional supplements has grown continuously. Often, the question is asked: "Can a pill or a capsule that contains important ingredients found in a plant have comparable benefits to eating the entire plant?" Most experts in the field and my own personal opinion is that the answer to this question is no. Eating adequate amounts of healthful food daily is preferable to taking a dietary supplement.

However, as I mentioned in Chapter 4, if we ask a second question: "Is there a role for dietary supplements to help ensure at least some of the benefits of soy for the greatest number of people?" the answer is a resounding yes.

I have been in practice for more than 20 years, and the number of my patients reaching menopause is increasing. Only a minority of them are willing to consider estrogen at all, and half of those will have stopped taking estrogen within 1 year. I found myself talking more and more about soy, offering recipes, and discussing other ways a patient can include soy in her diet. Many of my patients took my advice, but most did not eat soy every day, which would be the ideal way to get the most from soy's potential benefits. Others could not get used to the taste and would not eat it at all. I started wondering if a soy supplement for hot flashes would work, since I knew it would appeal to many women.

This need led me to help develop SoyCare Menopause—one of the first nutritional supplements intended to reduce hot flashes and the first soy supplement sold at mass merchandising outlets such as drugstores and chain stores. All of the soy ingredients are organically grown and GMO free (not genetically modified). Each capsule contains 25 mg of isoflavones. If 1 cap-

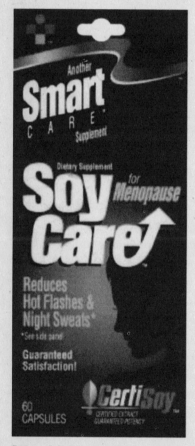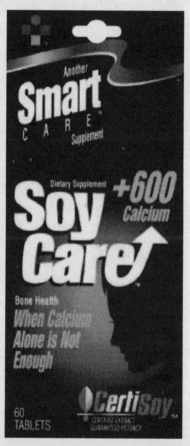

FIGURE 10-1.   SoyCare Supplements
SOURCE: Inverness Medical, Inc., Waltham, Massachusetts.

sule is taken twice daily, blood levels of the isoflavones are kept in a steady range throughout the day. This effect mimics the result of people eating the typical Asian diet. Since people who normally eat soy daily usually consume it in more than one meal, I think taking the supplement twice a day is important. I also insisted that if women weren't satisfied, they could get their money back for the product. Although this may sound like a promotion, I don't make any money from the sales of SoyCare. But I am able to reach a lot more women than I ever could by sitting in my office.

Since the development of SoyCare, other soy supplements have come on the market, including Healthy Woman, Caltrate 600 Plus Soy, and others.

Having said all this, what health benefits can we reasonably expect by taking soy supplements? I believe there are several.

- **Hot flashes.** Hot flashes respond well to soy nutritional supplements. They may not go away completely, but for the majority of women, hot flashes will be lowered by a significant amount and that may be enough to permit a good night's sleep.
- **Blood vessel elasticity.** Soy nutritional supplements also are able to keep blood vessel walls more elastic and that helps reduce hardening of the arteries.

TABLE 10-6. COMPARISON OF MAJOR SOY SUPPLEMENTS

Brand	Organic Soy	GMO Free	mg/ Capsule	Dosages/ Day
SoyCare Menopause	Yes	Yes	25	2
Healthy Woman	No	No	50	1
Caltrate 600 Plus Soy	No	No	50	1

- **Bone health.** Soy isoflavones, especially if combined with vitamin D and calcium, make a great way to combat bone loss. Soy is able to slow down the rate that calcium is lost from the bones. Of course, vitamin D helps absorb calcium, and calcium is the raw material that bones are made from.
- **Other.** The benefits of soy supplements in lowering cholesterol and lowering blood pressure are promising, but too little information is available to be certain that there is a specific benefit. The same is true of soy supplements and a possible preventive role against cancer.

COOKING WITH SOY

In this final section, I want to offer some specific ways to prepare soy foods. Try experimenting. Tofu is a great dessert ingredient. Whirled in the food processor or blender it turns into a creamy, smooth-textured ingredient for most traditional desserts, mild enough to take on chocolate, rum, butterscotch, or vanilla flavors. Sliced and grilled or baked soy is a wonderful appetizer or main course. Do not forget that soymilk can be substituted for anything you use milk for, from cereal and oatmeal to noodle kugel.

TABLE 10-7. SOYFOOD SUBSTITUTION CHART

Food	Soyfood Substitution	Serving Size	Fat Saved (grams)	Cholesterol Saved (grams)	Calories Saved
Ground beef, 85% lean	½ cup textured soy protein granules (plain or beef flavored), reconstituted	3 ounces, cooked	14	71	99
Cheddar cheese	Soy-based cheddar cheese	1 ounce	4	30	36
Dairy, 2% milk	Soymilk—lite or reduced-fat or reduced-fat reconstituted instant soymilk	8 ounces	3	18	20
Dairy, whole milk	Regular soymilk or regular reconstituted instant soymilk	8 ounces	4	33	7
Chicken breast, without skin, small chunks	Textured vegetable protein small chunks (chicken flavored) ½ cup rehydrated	3 ounces, cooked	3	77	58
Sour cream	Tofu sour cream	1 tablespoon	2.5	5	19
Egg (as a leavening agent in baking)	¼ cup silken "lite" firm tofu, mashed	Equivalent to 1 egg	4.5	213	53
Ricotta cheese, part skim	Tofu, firm, mashed to ricotta consistency	1 tablespoon	0	5	0

SOURCE: USDA Human Nutrition Service, Agriculture Handbook, #16–18, Composition of Food, Legumes and Legume Products; and Soyfoods Guide, distributed by the Soy Protein Partners. Stevens & Associates, Inc., 4816 N. Pennsylvania St., Indianapolis, IN 46205-1744.

Soy Recipes

Here are a few suggestions to help you get started. Some are compliments of friends, and the rest are my variations of existing recipes. Enjoy!

BREAKFAST

Soymilk French Toast

This simple variation of a breakfast staple is a delicious way to start your day with soy.

2 cups soymilk
2 tablespoons soy flour
½ teaspoon vanilla extract
Cooking spray
8 slices thick whole-grain bread

Combine soymilk, soy flour, and vanilla extract in a large bowl; stir with a wire whisk until blended. Spray a skillet or griddle with cooking spray; heat over medium-low heat. Dip bread into soymilk mixture, coating both sides evenly. Place each slice of bread in the skillet and cook for 2 to 3 minutes on each side or until golden brown. Top with maple syrup, applesauce, or fresh fruit.

Makes 4 servings (2 slices each serving)

Per serving: 254 calories, 39 grams carbohydrate, 10 grams protein, 6 grams fat, 0 grams saturated fat, 0 mg cholesterol, 375 mg sodium, 6 grams fiber

Whole Grain Pancakes

If you are looking for a simpler way to start your day, just reach into the pantry, pull out your favorite pancake mix, and substitute soymilk in equal measure to the milk or water you would normally use.

½ cup whole-wheat flour
¼ cup all-purpose flour
2 scoops soy-protein powder
2 teaspoons non-aluminum baking powder
¼ teaspoon salt
1⅓ cups soymilk
2 tablespoons soybean oil
Cooking spray

Mix together whole-wheat flour, all-purpose flour, soy-protein powder, baking powder, and salt in a medium bowl. Add soymilk and oil; stir just until blended. Spray a large skillet or griddle with cooking spray. Heat over medium-high heat until hot enough to evaporate a drop of water immediately upon contact.

Spoon batter by ¼-cup measures onto hot skillet or griddle. Cook until evenly covered with bubbles, about 2 minutes. Using a spatula, carefully turn over and cook for 1 to 2 minutes more, until lightly browned. Repeat with remaining batter. Spray the griddle or skillet again with cooking spray every time after making 2 pancakes.

Makes 4 servings (2 pancakes each serving)

Per serving: 198 calories, 19 grams carbohydrate, 17 grams protein, 9 grams fat, 1 gram saturated fat, 0 mg cholesterol, 362 mg sodium, 3 grams fiber

Soy Smoothie

It is easy to create your own breakfast smoothie recipe with different types of fruits. Try substituting vanilla soy yogurt for the soymilk for a different, great-tasting variation.

1 cup vanilla or plain soymilk
1 medium banana
¼ cup fresh or frozen unsweetened strawberries or ¼ cup fresh or frozen unsweetened peaches (optional)
5 ice cubes

Place all ingredients in a blender and process on medium speed for 1 minute or until smooth. Garnish with a strawberry and serve.

Makes 2 servings (1 cup each)

Per serving: 136 calories, 27 grams carbohydrate, 4 grams protein, 2 grams fat, 0 grams saturated fat, 0 mg cholesterol, 47 mg sodium, 2 grams fiber

LUNCH

Tacos with Beans

You can vary this recipe by using different flavored wraps and roll-ups instead of taco shells. If you are short on time or energy, try using a prepared taco seasoning mix instead of the spices.

1 cup textured vegetable protein or 1 pound tofu, crumbled
1 cup boiling water
2 8-ounce cans regular or no-salt-added tomato sauce (optional)
1 medium onion, chopped
2 cloves garlic, minced
2 teaspoons chili powder
1 teaspoon ground cumin
1 16-ounce can vegetarian refried beans
8 corn taco shells
Optional toppings: lettuce, tomatoes, salsa, grated soy cheese

Combine textured vegetable protein and boiling water in a large skillet or saucepan to rehydrate; stir and let stand for 5 to 10 minutes. If you use tofu, do not put in water. Stir in tomato sauce, onion, garlic, chili powder, and cumin. Cook over medium-high heat until mixture comes to a boil, stirring frequently. Reduce heat and simmer, uncovered, for 10 minutes or until the taco filling thickens. Heat refried beans in microwave. Place a layer of refried beans into each taco shell. Spoon ½ cup of taco filling on top. Add optional toppings and serve.

Makes 4 servings (2 tacos each serving)

Per serving: 328 calories, 49 grams carbohydrate, 22 grams protein, 9 grams fat, 1 gram saturated fat, 0 mg cholesterol, 690 mg sodium, 13 grams fiber

Meatless Sloppy Joes

Here is a new twist to an old favorite. You will not miss the meat.

1 cup textured vegetable protein
1 cup boiling water
1 16-ounce can sloppy Joe sauce
4 whole-wheat hamburger buns

Place the textured vegetable protein in a medium saucepan and pour the boiling water over it to rehydrate. Stir and let stand for 5 to 10 minutes. Stir in the sloppy Joe sauce and cook over medium heat for 3 to 4 minutes or until thoroughly heated. Spoon the mixture onto 4 buns and serve.

Makes 4 servings

Per serving: 246 calories, 42 grams carbohydrate, 18 grams protein, 3 grams fat, 0 grams saturated fat, 0 mg cholesterol, 852 mg sodium, 7 grams fiber

Grilled Marinated Tempeh

Lemon marinade is one of the best ways to enjoy tempeh. Try this one for an easy baked or grilled treat.

¼ cup fresh lemon juice
¼ cup olive oil
¼ teaspoon dried thyme
Black pepper to taste
16 ounces tempeh
1 large onion, sliced into rings
4 whole-wheat hamburger rolls
Lettuce and tomato slices for garnish

To prepare marinade, combine lemon juice, olive oil, thyme, and black pepper in a small bowl; set aside. Cut tempeh into slices. Using a steamer, steam tempeh for 15 minutes. Place tempeh and onions in a 2-quart casserole dish; pour the marinade over them. Refrigerate for at least 4 hours. Preheat oven to 400°F. Cover the casserole dish and bake for 30 to 35 minutes, or grill the tempeh and onions until thoroughly heated, basting frequently with marinade. Garnish with lettuce and tomato if desired. Serve hot on hamburger rolls.

Makes 4 servings

Per serving: 391 calories, 48 grams carbohydrate, 26 grams protein, 14 grams fat, 2 grams saturated fat, 0 mg cholesterol, 205 mg sodium, 9 grams fiber

DINNER

Sesame Tamari Tofu

This easy-to-prepare dish can also be served cold. (Compliments of Hari Kaur Khalsa)

Cooking spray
1 15-ounce package firm or extra-firm tofu
2 tablespoons tamari sauce
1 tablespoon crushed or whole sesame seeds
2 scallions, chopped

Spray a medium baking dish with cooking spray. Slice tofu into 10 to 12 slabs. Place in a gallon-size sealable plastic bag; add tamari sauce; seal bag, squeezing out air. Turn to coat tofu evenly. Refrigerate for at least 15 to 20 minutes, turning bag occasionally. Preheat oven to 350°F. Place tofu on baking dish; sprinkle with sesame seeds. Bake for 20 to 25 minutes or until lightly browned, turning once or twice for even browning. Top with scallions and serve hot.

Makes 4 servings

Per serving: 60 calories, 2 grams carbohydrate, 9 grams protein, 2 grams fat, 0 grams saturated fat, 0 mg cholesterol, 608 mg sodium, 0 grams fiber

Tofu Lasagna Casserole

Here's a healthy way to improve upon one of my favorite Italian dishes. Crumbled tofu makes an excellent substitute for ricotta cheese, and soy mozzarella and soy Parmesan take the place of the dairy products. Mangia!

Cooking spray
1½ pounds soft tofu, crumbled
10 large mushrooms, chopped
1½ teaspoons dried oregano
1½ teaspoons dried basil
2½ cups prepared pasta sauce
9 lasagna noodles, uncooked

2 cups commercially prepared béchamel sauce
8 ounces shredded soy mozzarella-flavor cheese
¼ cup grated soy Parmesan-flavor cheese
¼ cup water

Preheat oven to 350°F. Spray a 9 × 13-inch baking pan with cooking spray. Combine tofu, mushrooms, oregano, and basil in a large bowl; mix well. Spread about ½ cup of pasta sauce in the bottom of the baking pan. Layer in order as follows: 3 uncooked noodles, ½ cup pasta sauce, half of the tofu mixture, 1 cup béchamel sauce, and half of the soy mozzarella cheese. For the next layer: add 3 uncooked noodles, ½ cup pasta sauce, remaining tofu mixture, remaining béchamel sauce, and remaining soy mozzarella cheese. Top with the last 3 uncooked noodles and 1 cup pasta sauce. Sprinkle top of lasagna with soy Parmesan cheese. Pour the water into a corner of the pan; cover baking pan with foil and bake for 45 to 50 minutes or until noodles are tender and edges are bubbling. Let stand for 5 to 10 minutes before serving.

Makes 8 servings

Per serving: 383 calories, 38 grams carbohydrate, 22 grams protein, 16 grams fat, 4 grams saturated fat, 16 mg cholesterol, 1,601 mg sodium, 3 grams fiber

Soy Mozzarella Pizza

If you like pizza, you'll love this soy-based taste-alike. And you will be getting all the wonderful benefits of soy. For an exciting variation, add soy pepperoni, sliced mushrooms, black olives, and/or cooked soy sausage.

Cooking spray
Cornmeal for dusting
1 package active dry yeast
1 cup warm water
2 tablespoons olive oil
2 cups all-purpose flour
½ cup soy flour
½ teaspoon salt
2 cups prepared pasta sauce
1 tablespoon Italian seasoning
10 to 12 ounces shredded soy mozzarella-flavor cheese

Preheat oven to 450°F. Spray a 14-inch pizza pan with cooking spray and dust with cornmeal. Combine yeast, warm water, and olive oil in a small bowl. Combine all-purpose flour, soy flour, and salt in a large bowl; stir in the yeast mixture using a rubber spatula to make a soft dough. Place the dough on a floured surface and knead for 5 minutes or until dough becomes smooth and elastic. Cover with clear plastic wrap and allow to sit for about 10 minutes. Using your hands, flatten and shape dough. Place onto pizza pan. Top with pasta sauce, Italian seasoning, and cheese. Bake for 10 to 12 minutes or until the pizza crust is crisp and cheese is bubbling.

Makes 6 servings (1 slice each serving)

Per serving: 370 calories, 48 grams carbohydrate, 19 grams protein, 15 grams fat, 1 gram saturated fat, 0 mg cholesterol, 1,293 mg sodium, 4 grams fiber

Fresh Green Soybeans

Enjoy this side dish with a dash of your favorite herbs and/or spices. Rosemary and garlic work well together.

1 pound fresh soybeans in the pod
4 cups boiling water
1 cup cold water
⅛ teaspoon salt

Place soybeans in a large saucepan; add boiling water until soybeans are covered. Let stand for 5 minutes. Drain water. Break the pods open and remove the beans; discard the pods. Replace the beans into the same saucepan; add cold water and bring to a gentle boil over medium-high heat for 15 to 20 minutes or until beans are tender. Sprinkle with salt and serve hot.

Makes 3 servings (½ cup each serving)

Per serving: 127 calories, 10 grams carbohydrate, 11 grams protein, 6 grams fat, 1 gram saturated fat, 0 mg cholesterol, 110 mg sodium, 4 grams fiber

Soy Cookbooks

- *The Art of Tofu* by Akasha Richmond. Torrance, Calif: Morinaga Publishers; 1997.
- *Soy! Soy! Soy!* by Jeanette Parsons Egan. Tucson, Ariz: Fisher Books; 1999.
- *The Whole Soy Cookbook* by Patricia Greenberg and Helen Newton Hartung. New York: Three Rivers Press; 1998.
- *The Soy Zone: 101 Delicious and Easy-to-Prepare Recipes* by Barry Sears. New York: Regan Books; 2000.
- *Tofu and Soyfoods Cookery* by Peter Golbitz. Summertown, Tenn: Book Publishing Company; 1998.
- *The Complete Soy Cookbook: 180 Gourmet Recipes for Great Taste and Good Health* by Paulette Mitchell. New York: Hungry Minds, Inc.; 1997.
- *The Soy Gourmet* by Robin Peterson. New York: Dutton; 1998.
- *New Soy Cookbook: Tempting Recipes for Soybeans, Soymilk, Tofu, Tempeh, Miso and Soy Sauce* by Lorna J. Sass and Jonelle Weaver. San Francisco: Chronicle Books; 1998.
- *The Soy of Cooking: Easy to Make Vegetarian, Low-Fat, Fat-Free, and Antioxidant-Rich Gourmet Recipes* by Marie Oser. New York: John Wylie & Sons; 1996.
- *The Book of Tofu* by William Shurtleff and Akiko Aoyagi. Berkeley, Calif: Ten Speed Press; 1998.

Soy Recipes and Foods Web Sites

- *Dixie Diner*. Find soy-based foods that taste like the real thing. Lots of recipes and health information. (*www.dixiediner.com*)
- *Vegging Out—Soy Recipes*. Learn how to make scones, hummus, brownies, and soups. (*www.execpc.com/~veggie/recipes.html*)

- *Iowa Soy.* Soy recipes, cooking tips, and health benefits. (*www.iowasoy.com*)
- *StratSoy—Nutrition and Recipes.* Articles on the health benefits of soy, links to soy foods, and soy recipes. (*www.stratsoy.uiuc.edu/indexes/Nutrition.html*)
- *Vitasoy USA, Inc.* Recipes for a whole variety of soy-based foods and links to soy products. (*www.vitasoy-usa.com*)
- *Soy.com—Recipes.* Recipes for soy-based appetizers, side dishes, soups, entrées, salads, and desserts using soy and tofu products. (*www.soy.com/recipes.html*)
- *Vegetarian Times—Soy-Based Recipes.* A collection of international recipes such as moussaka and chimichangas based on soy. (*www.findarticles.com/m0820/2000Feb/59269772/p1/article.jhtml*)
- *Simply Soy Bread Recipes.* Recipes replace the flour in yeast breads with soy flour. Find muffins, bread machines, and fruit goods. (*www.soyfoods.com/SimplySoy/Breads/Breads.html*)
- *Simply Soy Sandwich Recipes.* Learn how to make meatless sandwiches. Mock egg salad, grilled soy cheese, and barbecued tempeh. (*www.soyfoods.com/SimplySoy/Sandwiches/Sandwiches.html*)
- *Eden Foods, Inc.* Find recipes and soy-based foods. (*www.edensoy.com*)
- *Genisoy Products.* Information on soy protein bars, drinks, powders, and recipes. (*www.genisoy.com*)

NOTES

INTRODUCTION

1. FDA Talk Paper. FDA Approves New Health Claim for Soy Protein and Coronary Heart Disease. T 99–48. October 20, 1999.
2. North American Menopause Society. *www.menopause.org/news.*

CHAPTER 1

1. Kato I, Toniolo P, Akmedkhanov A, et al. Prospective study of factors influencing the onset of natural menopause. *J Clin Epidemiol.* 1998;51:1271–1276.
2. Uzilelli ML, Guarducci S, Lapi E, et al. Premature ovarian failure (POF) and fragile X premutation females: from POF to fragile X carrier identification, from fragile X diagnosis to POF association data. *Am J Med Genet.* 1999;84:300–303.
3. Shandler N. *Estrogen the Natural Way.* New York: Villard Press; 1997.
4. Seibel MM, Khalsa HK. *A Woman's Book of Yoga.* New York: Penguin, Putnam, Avery Press; 2002.
5. Gittleman AL. *Before the Change.* San Francisco: Harper; 1999.
6. Quoted in Gray FD. The third age. *The New Yorker.* February 26 and March 4, 1996:191.

7. Maroulis GB. Aging and Reproduction. In: Seibel MM, ed. *Infertility: A Comprehensive Text*. Norwalk, Conn: Appleton & Lange; 1997.

8. Centers for Disease Control. *www.cdc.gov/nccdphp/drh/art*.

9. Bar-Ami S, Seibel MM. Oocyte development and meiosis in humans. In: Seibel, MM, ed. *Infertility: A Comprehensive Text*. Norwalk, Conn: Appleton & Lange; 1997.

10. Faddy MF, Gosden RG, Gougeon A, et al. Accelerated disappearance of ovarian follicles in mid-life: implications for forecasting menopause. *Hum Reprod*. 1992;7:1342–1346.

11. Minkin MJ, Wright CV. *What Every Woman Needs to Know About Menopause*. New Haven, Conn: Yale University Press; 1996.

12. Shideler SE, DeVane GW, Kalra PS, Benirschke K, Lasley BI. Ovarian pituitary hormone interactions during the perimenopause. *Maturitas*. 1989;11(4):331–339.

13. Cauley JA, Gutal JP, Kuller LH, LeDonne D, Powell JG. The epidemiology of serum sex hormones in postmenopausal women. *Am J Epidemiol*. 1989;129(6):1120–1131.

14. Adashi EY. The climacteric ovary as a functional gonadotropin-driven androgen-producing gland. *Fertil Steril*. 1994;62:20–27.

15. Love SM, Lindsey K. *Dr. Susan Love's Hormone Book*. New York: Random House; 1997.

16. Seibel MM, Freeman MG, Graves WL. Hysterectomy for carcinoma in situ and sexual function. *Gynecol Oncol*. 1981;11:195–199.

17. Thomas TM, Plymat KR, Blannin J, Meade TW. Prevalence of urinary incontinence. *Br Med J*. 1980;281:143–145.

18. DeLancey JOL. Structural support of the urethra as it relates to stress urinary incontinence: the hammock hypothesis. *Am J Obstet Gynecol*. 1994;170:1713–1723.

19. *Menopause Guidebook*. North American Menopause Society 2001:16. *www.menopause.org*.

20. *AMA Essential Guide to Menopause.* American Medical Association. New York: Pocket Books; 1998.

21. Skeleton DA, Young A, Greig CA, Malbut KE. Effects of resistance training on strength, power, and selected functional abilities of women aged 75 and older. *J Am Geriatr Soc.* 1995;43:1081–1087.

22. Abrahms P, Freeman R, Anderstrom C, et al. Tolterodine, a new antimuscarinic agent as effective but better tolerated than oxybutynin in patients with overactive bladder. *Br J Urol.* 1998;81:801–810.

23. Wein AJ, Rovner ES. The overactive bladder: an overview for primary care health providers. *Int J Fertil Womens Med.* 1999;44:56–66.

24. Nygaard I. Prevention of exercise incontinence with mechanical devices. *J Repro Med.* 1995;40(2):89–94.

25. Howard D, DeLancey JOL. The stress continence control system. *Postgrad Obstet Gynecol.* 1999;19(7):1–6.

26. *Second Task Force on Female Sexuality During the Menopause.* OBG Management. May 2000.

27. US Bureau of the Census: Current Population Reports, Special Studies. 65+ in the United States. Washington, DC: U.S. Government Printing Office. P23–190.

28. Kalb C. A little help in the bedroom. *Newsweek.* Special Issue. Spring/Summer 1999:38–39.

29. Russell RM. The aging process as a modifier of metabolism. *Am J Clin Nutr.* 2000;72(suppl):529S–532S.

30. Roberts SB, Russ P, Heyman MB, et al. Control of food intake in older men. *JAMA.* 1994;272:601–606.

31. Hurwitz A, Brady A, Schaal E, Samloff I, Delon J, Ruhl C. Gastric acidity in older adults. *JAMA.* 1997;278: 659–662.

32. Mort JR, Lemon MD. Smoking cessation and the depressed patient. *US Pharmacist.* 2000;25(3):28–38.

33. Holte A. Influences of natural menopause on health complaints: a prospective study of healthy Norwegian women. *Maturitas*. 1992;14:1127–1141.

34. Kaufert PA, Gilbert P, Tate R. The Manitoba Project: a reexamination of the link between menopause and depression. *Maturitas*. 1992;14:143–155.

35. New England Research Institute, Inc. *Women and Their Health in Massachusetts: Final Report*. Watertown, Mass; 1991.

36. Greenlee RT, Murray T, Bolden S, Wingo PA. Cancer statistics 2000. *CA Cancer J Clin*. 2000;50(1):7–33.

37. Grady D, Rubin SM, Petitti DB, et al. Hormone therapy to prevent disease and prolong life in postmenopausal women. *Ann Intern Med*. 1992;117:1016–1037.

38. Cooper GM. *Elements of Human Cancer*. Sudbury, Mass: Jones and Bartlett; 1992.

39. Bernstein L, Henderson BE, Hanisch R, Sullivan-Halley J, Ross RK. Physical exercise and reduced risk of breast cancer in young women. *JNCI* 1994;86(18):1403–1408.

40. Underwood A. *Newsweek*. Special Issue. Spring/Summer 1999:44.

41. Greenlee RT, et al. Cancer statistics 2000. *CA Cancer J Clin*. 2000;50(1):7–33.

42. Greenlee RT, Hill-Harmon MB, Murray T, Thun M. Cancer statistics, 2001. *CA Cancer J Clin*. 2001;51:15–36.

CHAPTER 2

1. Oddens BJ, Boulet MJ, Lehert P, et al. A study on the use of medication for climacteric complaints in Western Europe—II. *Maturitas*. 1994;19:1–12.

2. MacLennan AH, Wilson DH, Taylor AW. Hormone replacement therapy, prevalence, compliance, and the "healthy woman" notion. *Climacteric*. 1998;1–42.

3. White E, Velentgas P, Mandelson MT, et al. Variation in

mammographic density by the time in menstrual cycle among women aged 40–49 years. *JNCI.* 1998;90:906–910.

4. Stomper PC, D'Souza DJ, DiNitto PA, Arredondo MA. Analysis of parenchymal density on mammograms in 1353 women 25–79 years old. *AJR.* 1996;167:1261–1265.

5. Persson I, Thurfjell E, Holmberg L. Effect of estrogen and estrogen-progestin replacement regimens on mammographic breast parenchymal density. *J Clin Oncol.* 1997;15:3201–3207.

6. Harvey JA. The mammogram in menopause: how hormones influence imaging. *Menopausal Medicine.* Spring 2000; 8:5–9.

7. Laya MB, Larson EB, Taplin SH, White E. Effect of estrogen replacement therapy on the specificity and sensitivity of screening mammography. *JNCI.* 1996;88:643–649.

8. Wilson RA. *Feminine Forever.* New York: M Evans and Company; 1966.

9. Simon J, Klaiber E, Wiita B, et al. Differential effects of estrogen-androgen and estrogen-only therapy on vasomotor symptoms, gonadotropin secretion, and endogenous androgen bioavailability in postmenopausal women. *Menopause.* 1999;6:138–146.

10. Hammar M, Ekblad S, Lonnberg B, et al. Postmenopausal women without previous or current vasomotor symptoms do not flush after abruptly abandoning estrogen replacement therapy. *Maturitas.* 1999;31:117–122.

11. Matkovic V. Nutrition genetics and skeletal development. *J Am Coll Nutr.* 1996;15:556–561.

12. Lindsay R, Hart DM, Aitken JM, et al. Long-term prevention of postmenopausal osteoporosis by oestrogen. Evidence for an increased bone mass after delayed onset of oestrogen treatment. *Lancet.* 1976;1:1038–1041.

13. Greendale GA, Wells B, Marcus R, Barrett-Connor E. Postmenopausal Estrogen/Progestin Interventions Trial Investigators. *Arch Intern Med.* 2000;160:3065–3071.

14. Weiss NS, Ure CL, Ballard JH, et al. Decreased risk of fractures of the hip and lower forearm with postmenopausal use of estrogen. *N Engl J Med.* 1980;303:1195–1198.

15. Ettinger B. Personal perspective on low-dose estrogen therapy for postmenopausal women. *Menopause.* 1999;6: 273–276.

16. Weiss SR, Ellman H, Kolker M. A randomized controlled trial of four doses of transdermal estradiol for preventing postmenopausal bone loss. Transdermal Estradiol Investigators Group. *Obstet Gynecol.* 1999;94:330–336.

17. Delmas PD, Pornel B, Felsenberg D, et al. A dose-ranging trial of matrix transdermal 17 beta-estradiol for the prevention of bone loss in early postmenopausal women. International Study Group. *Bone.* 1999;24:517–523.

18. Mishell DR. Evaluating the benefits and risks of hormone replacement therapy. *Ob Gyn News.* December 2000; suppl:1–11.

19. Schiff I, Parson AB. *Menopause.* New York: Times Books; 1996:142.

20. Birkenfeld L, Yemini M, Kase NG, et al. Menopause-related oral alveolar bone resorption: a review of relatively unexplored consequences of estrogen deficiency. *Menopause.* 1999;6:129–133.

21. Reinhardt RA, Payne JB, Maze CA, et al. Influence of estrogen and osteopenia/osteoporosis on clinical periodontitis in postmenopausal women. *J Periodontol.* 1999;70:823–828.

22. Lindsay R, Tohme JF. Estrogen treatment of patients with established postmenopausal osteoporosis. *Obstet Gynecol.* 1990;76:290–295.

23. Recker RR, Davies KM, Dowd RM, Heaney RP. The effect of low-dose continuous estrogen and progesterone therapy with calcium and vitamin D on bone in elderly women. A randomized, controlled trial. *Ann Intern Med.* 1999;130: 897–904.

24. Resnick NM. Urinary incontinence. *Lancet*. 1995;346: 94–99.

25. DeLancey JOL. Structural support of the urethra as it relates to stress urinary incontinence: the hammock hypothesis. *Am J Obstet Gynecol*. 1994;170:1713–1723.

26. Nygaard IE, Thompson FL, Svengalis SL, Albright JP. Urinary incontinence in elite nulliparous athletes. *Obstet Gynecol*.1994;84:183–187.

27. Hillier SL, Lau RJ. Vaginal microflora in postmenopausal women who have not received estrogen replacement therapy. *Clin Infect Dis*. 1997;25(suppl 2):S123–S126.

28. Bachmann GA. The clinical platform for the 17 beta-estradiol vaginal releasing ring. *Am J Obstet Gynecol*. 1998;178: S257–S260.

29. Cordoza L, Bachmann G, McClish D, et al. Meta-analysis of estrogen therapy in the management of urogenital atrophy in postmenopausal women: second report of the Hormones and Urogenital Therapy Committee. *Obstet Gynecol*. 1998;92: 722–727.

30. Eriksen B. A randomized, open, parallel-group study on the preventive effect of an estradiol-releasing vaginal ring (Estring) on recurrent urinary tract infections in post-menopausal women. *Am J Obstet Gynecol*. 1999;180: 1072–1079.

31. Berman KF, Schmidt PJ, Rubinow DR, et al. Modulation of cognition-specific cortical activity by gonadal steroids: a positron-emission tomography study in women. *Proc Natl Acad Sci USA*. 1997;94:8836–8841.

32. Henderson VW. Estrogen, cognition, and a woman's risk of Alzheimer's disease. *Am J Med*. 1997;103(suppl 3A): 11–18.

33. Brinton RD, Tran J, Proffitt P, et al. 17-beta-estradiol enhances the outgrowth and survival of neocortical neurons in culture. *Neurochem Res*. 1997;22:1339–1351.

34. CarranzaLira S, Valentino-Figueroa M. Estrogen therapy for depression in postmenopausal women. *Int J Gynaecol Obstet.* 1999;65:35–38.

35. Hogervorst E, Boshuisen M, Riedel W, et al. Curt P. Richter Award. The effect of hormone replacement on cognitive function in elderly women. *Psychoneuroendocrinology.* 1999;24:43–68.

36. Van Duijin CM. Hormone replacement therapy and Alzheimer's disease. *Maturitas.* 1999;31:201–205.

37. Fettes I. Migraine in the menopause. *Neurology.* 1999; 53(suppl 1):S3–S13.

38. Ogueta SB, Schwartz SD, Yamashita CK, et al. Estrogen receptor in the human eye: influence of gender and age on gene expression. *Invest Ophthalmol Vis Sci.* 1999;40: 1906–1911.

39. Grodstein F, Martinez ME, Platz EA, et al. Postmenopausal hormone use and risk for colon cancer and adenoma. *Ann Intern Med.* 1998;128:705–712.

40. Collins JA, Schlesselman JJ. Hormone replacement therapy and endometrial cancer. In: Lobo RA, ed. *Treatment of the Postmenopausal Woman: Basic and Clinical Aspects.* 2nd ed. Philadelphia: Lippincott, Williams & Wilkins; 1999:503–511.

41. Effects of hormone replacement therapy on endometrial histology in postmenopausal women. The Postmenopausal Estrogen/Progestin Interventions (PEPI) Trial. The Writing Group for the PEPI Trial. *JAMA.* 1996;275:370–375.

42. Gruber DM, Wagner G, Kurz C, et al. Endometrial cancer after combined hormone replacement therapy. *Maturitas.* 1999;31:237–240.

43. Rodriguez C, Patel AV, Calle EE, Jacob EJ, Thun MJ. Estrogen replacement therapy and ovarian cancer mortality in a large study of US women. *JAMA.* 2001;285: 1460–1465.

44. Grodstein F, Stampfer MJ, Goldhaber SZ, et al. Prospective study of exogenous hormones and risk of pulmonary embolism in women. *Lancet.* 1996;348:983–987.

45. Jick H, Derby LE, Myers MW, et al. Risk of hospital admission for idiopathic venous thromboembolism among users of postmenopausal oestrogens. *Lancet.* 1996;348:981–983.

46. Daly E, Vessey MP, Hawkins MM, et al. Risk of venous thromboembolism in users of hormone replacement therapy. *Lancet.* 1996;348:977–980.

47. Oger E, Scarabin PY. Assessment of the risk for venous thrombosis among users of hormone replacement therapy. *Drugs Aging.* 1999;14:55–61.

48. Gallup Poll for Walnut Marketing Board. National Center for Health Statistics; 1995.

49. Brinton LA, Hoover RN. Estrogen replacement therapy and endometrial cancer risk: unresolved issues. The Endometrial Cancer Collaborative Group. *Obstet Gynecol.* 1993;81:265–271.

50. Schairer C, Lubin J, Troisi R, Sturgeon S, Brinton L, Hoover R. Menopausal estrogen and estrogen-progestin replacement therapy and breast cancer risk. *JAMA.* 2000;283:485–491.

51. Magnusson C, Baron JA, Correia N, Bergstrom R, Adami O, Persson I. Breast cancer risk following long-term oestrogen-progestin-replacement therapy. *Int J Cancer Inst.* 1999;81:339–344.

52. Ross RK, Paganini-Hill A, Wan PC, Pike MC. Effect of hormone replacement therapy on breast cancer risk: estrogen versus estrogen plus progestin. *JNCI.* 2000;92 328–332.

53. Magnusson C, Baron JA, Correia N, Bergstrom R, Adami O, Persson I. Breast cancer risk following long-term oestrogen-progestin-replacement therapy. *Int J Cancer Inst.* 1999;81:339–344.

54. Colditz GA, Hankinson SE, Hunter DJ, et al. The use of estrogens and progestins and the risk of breast cancer in postmenopausal women. *N Engl J Med.* 1995;332:1589.

55. Persson I, Weiderpass E, Bergkvist L, Bergstrom R, Schairer C. Risks of breast and endometrial cancer after estrogen and estrogen-progestin replacement. *Cancer Causes Control.* 1999;10:253–260.

56. Kaufman DW, Miller DR, Rosenberg L, et al. Noncontraceptive estrogen use and the risk of breast cancer. *JAMA.* 1984;252:63–67.

57. Ewertz M. Influence of non-contraceptive exogenous and endogenous sex hormones on breast cancer risk in Denmark. *Int J Cancer.* 1988;42:832–838.

58. Bergkvist L, Adami H-O, Persson I, Hoover R, Schairer C. The risk of breast cancer after estrogen and estrogen-progestin replacement. *N Engl J Med.* 1989;321:293.

59. Yang CP, Daling JR, Band PR, Gallagher RP, White E, Weiss NS. Noncontraceptive hormone use and risk of breast cancer. *Cancer Causes Control.* 1992;3:475.

60. Stanfork JL, Weiss NS, Voight LF, Daling JR, Habel LA, Rossing MA. Combined estrogen and progestin hormone replacement therapy in relation to risk of breast cancer in middle-aged women. *JAMA.* 1995;274:137.

61. Newcomb PA, Longnecker MP, Storer BE, et al. Long-term hormone replacement therapy and risk of breast cancer in postmenopausal women. *Am J Epidemiol.* 1995;142:788–795.

62. La Vecchia C, Negri E, Franceschi S. Hormone replacement therapy and breast cancer risk; a cooperative Italian study. *Br J Cancer.* 1995;72:244–248.

63. Collaborative Group on Hormonal Factors in Breast Cancer. Breast cancer and hormone replacement therapy: collaborative reanalysis of data from 51 epidemiological studies of 52,705 women with breast cancer and 108,411 women without breast cancer. *Lancet.* 1997;350:1047–1059.

64. Brinton LA, Brogan DR, Coates RJ, Swanson CA, Potischman N, Stanford JL. Breast cancer risk among women under 55 years of age by joint effects of usage of oral contraceptives and hormone replacement therapy. *Menopause.* 1998;5:145–151.

65. Thomas HV, Key TJ, Allen DS, et al. Re: reversal relation between body mass and endogenous estrogen concentrations with menopausal status. *JNCI.* 1997;89:396–398.

66. Cauley JA, Lucas FL, Kuller LH, Stone K, Browner W, Cummings SR. Elevated serum estradiol and testosterone concentrations are associated with a high risk for breast cancer. *Ann Intern Med.* 1999;130:270–277.

67. Henderson BE, Ross RK, Judd HL, Krailo MD, Pike MC. Do regular ovulatory cycles increase breast cancer risk? *Cancer.* 1985;56:1206–1208.

68. Clemons M, Goss P. Estrogen and the risk of breast cancer. *N Engl J Med.* 2001;344:276–285.

69. Hunt K, Vessey M, McPherson K. Mortality in a cohort of long-term users of hormone replacement therapy: an updated analysis. *Br J Obstet Gynaecol.* 1990;97:1080.

70. Grodstein F, Stampfer MJ, Colditz GA, et al. Postmenopausal hormone therapy and mortality. *N Engl J Med.* 1997;336:1769–1775.

71. Schairer C, Gail M, Byrne C, et al. Estrogen replacement therapy and breast cancer survival in a large screening study. *JNCI.* 1999;91:264–270.

72. Jernstrom H, Frenander J, Ferno M, Olson H. Hormone replacement therapy before breast cancer diagnosis significantly reduces the overall death rate compared with never-use among 984 breast cancer patients. *Br J Cancer.* 1999;80:1453–1458.

73. Speroff L. A clinician's response to the epidemiological data linking postmenopausal estrogen-progestin therapy with an increased risk of breast cancer. *Menopausal Medicine.* 2000;8(1):1–5.

74. Schairer C, Gail M, Byrne C, et al. Estrogen replacement therapy and breast cancer survival in a large screening study. *JNCI.* 1999;91:264–270.

75. Vassilopoulou-Sellin R, Asmar L, Hortobagyi GN, et al. Estrogen replacement therapy after localized breast cancer: clinical outcome of 319 women followed prospectively. *J Clin Oncol.* 1999;17:1482–1487.

76. Ganz PA, Greendale GA, Kahn B, et al. Are older breast carcinoma survivors willing to take hormone replacement therapy? *Cancer.* 1999;86:814–820.

77. Ferguson DP, Anderson TJ. Morphological evaluation of cell turnover in relation to menstrual cycle in the "resting" human breast. *Br J Cancer.* 1988;44:177.

78. Spicer DV, Krecker EA, Pike M. The endocrine prevention of breast cancer. *Cancer Invest.* 1995;13:495–504.

79. Ross RK, Paganini-Hill A, Wan PC, et al. Effect of hormone replacement therapy on breast cancer risk: estrogen versus estrogen plus progestin. *JNCI.* 2000;92:328–332.

80. Schairer C, Lubin J, Troisi R, et al. Menopausal estrogen and estrogen-progestin replacement therapy and breast cancer risk. *JAMA.* 2000;283:485–491.

81. Helzlsouer KJ, Alberg AJ, Bush TL, Longcope C, Gordon GB, Comstock GW. A prospective study of endogenous hormones and breast cancer. *Cancer Detect Prev.* 1994;18:79.

82. Chang K-J, Lee TTY, Linarez-Cruz G, Fournier S, de LigniEres B. Influences of percutaneous administration of estradiol and progesterone on human breast epithelial cell cycle in vivo. *Fertil Steril.* 1995;63:7857–7891.

83. Kester HA, van der Leede BM, van der Saag PT, van der Burg B. Novel progesterone target genes identified by an improved differential display technique suggest that progestin-induced growth inhibition of breast cancer cells coincides with enhancement of differentiation. *J Biol Chem.* 1997; 272:16637–16643.

84. American Heart Association. About women, heart disease and stroke. Available at: *www.americanheart.org/statistics/02about*.

85. Wagner JD. Rationale for hormone replacement therapy in atherosclerosis prevention. *J Reprod Med*. 2000;45:245–268.

86. Rosano GM, Panina G. Cardiovascular pharmacology of hormone replacement therapy. *Drugs Aging*. 1999;15:219–234.

87. Weintraub M, Grosskopf I, Charach G, et al. Hormone replacement therapy enhances postprandial lipid metabolism in postmenopausal women. *Metabolism*. 1999;48:1193–1196.

88. The writing group for the PEPI Trial. Effects of estrogen or estrogen/progestin regimens on heart disease risk factors in postmenopausal women: the Postmenopausal Estrogen/Progestin Interventions (PEPI) Trial. *JAMA*. 1995;273:199–208.

89. Collins P, Rossano GMC, Sarrel PM, et al. Estradiol 17 attenuates acetyl-choline induced coronary arterial constriction in women but not in men with coronary heart disease. *Circulation*. 1995;92:24–30.

90. Hanke H, Hanke S, Bruck B, et al. Inhibition of the protective effect of estrogen by progesterone in experimental atherosclerosis. *Atherosclerosis*. 1996;121:129–138.

91. Hulley S, Grady D, Bush T, et al. Randomized trial of estrogen plus progestin for secondary prevention of coronary heart disease in postmenopausal women. *JAMA*. 1998;280:605–613.

92. Herrington DM, Reboussin DM, Brosnihan KB, et al. Effects of estrogen replacement on the progression of coronary artery atherosclerosis. *N Engl J Med*. 2000;343:522–529.

93. Statement from Claude Lenfant, MD, NHLBI director, on preliminary trends in the Women's Health Initiative. National Heart, Lung, and Blood Institute press release. April 3, 2000.

94. Gotto AM. Statin therapy: Where are we? Where do we go next? *J Am Col Cardiol*. 2001;87:13B–18B.

95. *Tufts University Health & Nutrition Letter.* June 2001;19:6.

96. Casper RF, MacLusky NJ, Vanin C, et al. Rationale for estrogen with interrupted progestin as a new low-dose hormonal replacement therapy. *J Soc Gynecol Invest.* 1996;3: 225–234.

97. Reiss U, Zucker M. *Natural Hormone Balance for Women.* New York: Pocket Books; 2001.

98. Lemon HM. Estriol prevention of mammary carcinoma induced by 7,12-dimethylbenzanthracene and procarbazine. *Cancer Res.* 1975;35(5):1341–1353.

99. Lemon HM. Pathophysiologic considerations in the treatment of menopausal patients with oestrogens; the role of oestriol in the prevention of mammary carcinoma. *Acta Endocrinol (Copenhagen).* 1980;233(suppl):17–27.

100. Dickinson LE, MacMahon B, Cole P, Brown JB. Estrogen profiles of oriental and caucasian women in Hawaii. *N Eng J Med.* 1974;291:1211–1213.

101. Key TJ, Wang DY, Brown JB, et al. A prospective study of urinary oestrogen excretion and breast cancer risk. *Br J Cancer.* 1996;73(12):1615–1619.

102. Whitehead MI. Prevention of endometrial abnormalities. *Acta Obstet Gynecol Scand.* 1986;134(suppl):81–91.

103. Yang TS, Tsan SH, Chang SP, Ng HT. Efficacy and safety of estriol replacement therapy for climacteric women. *Chung Hua I Hsueh Tsa Chih (Taipei).* May 1995;55(5): 386–391.

104. Luciano AA, Miller BE, Schoenenfeld MJ, Schaser RJ. Effects of estrone sulfate alone or with medroxyprogesterone acetate on serum lipoprotein levels in postmenopausal women. *Obstet Gynecol.* 2001;97:101–108.

105. Foidart JM, Beliard A, Hedon B, et al. Impact of percutaneous oestradiol gels in postmenopausal hormone replacement therapy on clinical symptoms and endometrium. *Br J Obstet Gynaecol.* 1997;104(3):305–310.

106. Palacios S, Menendez C, Jurado AR, Vargas JC. Effects of percutaneous oestradiol (Estreva) versus oral oestrogens on bone density. *Maturitas*. 1994;20:209–213.

107. Reiss U, Zucker M. *Natural Hormone Balance for Women*. New York: Pocket Books; 2001:99–142.

108. Assikis VJ, Jordan VC. A realistic assessment of the association between tamoxifen and endometrial cancer. *Endocr Rel Cancers*. 1995;2:1–7.

109. Gottardis MM, Robinson SP, Satyaswaroop PG, et al. Contrasting actions of tamoxifen on endometrial and breast tumor growth in the athymic mouse. *Cancer Res*. 1988;48:812–815.

110. Powles TJ, Hickish T, Kanis JA, et al. Effect of tamoxifen on bone mineral density measured by dual-energy x-ray absorptiometry in healthy premenopausal and postmenopausal women. *J Clin Oncol*. 1996;14:78–84.

111. Raloxifene package insert. International Multicenter Study. Indianapolis: Eli Lilly and Company; 1998.

112. Davies GC, Huster WJ, Lu Y, et al. Adverse events reported by postmenopausal women in controlled trials with raloxifene. *Obstet Gynecol*. 1999;130:545–553.

CHAPTER 3

1. Seibel MM. The role of nutrition and nutritional supplements in women's health. *Fertil Steril*. 1999;72:579–591.

2. Blusztajn JK. Choline, a vital amine. *Science*. 1998;281:794–795.

3. Setchell KDR. Phytoestrogens: the biochemistry, physiology, and implications for human health of soy isoflavones. *Am J Clin Nutr*. 1998;68(suppl):1333S–1346S.

4. Simoons FJ. *Food in China. A Cultural and Historical Inquiry*. Boca Raton, Ann Arbor, Boston: CRC Press Inc.; 1991.

5. Messina M, Messina V, Setchell K. *The Simple Soybean and*

Your Health. Garden City Park, NY: Avery Publishing Group; 1994.

6. Council for Agricultural Science and Technology. How much land can ten billion people spare for nature? Ames, Iowa: Council for Agricultural Science and Technology, 1994; Talk Force Report no. 121.

7. Rogers SG. Biotechnology and the soybean. *Am J Clin Nutr.* 1998;68(suppl):1330S–1332S.

8. Greenberg P, Hartung HN. *The Whole Soy Cookbook.* New York: Three Rivers Press; 1998.

9. Baker ME. Evolution of regulation of steroid-mediated intercellular communication in vertebrates: insights from flavonoids, signals that mediate plant-rhizobia symbiosis. *J Steroid Biochem Mol Biol.* 1992;41:301–308.

10. National Research Council. *Recommended daily allowances.* 10th edition. Washington, DC: National Academy Press; 1989.

11. Stabler SP, Marcel PD, Podell ER, Allen RH, Savage DG, Lindenbaum J. Elevation of total homocysteine in the serum of patients with cobalamin or folate deficiency detected by capillary gas chromatography. *J Clin Invest.* 1988;114:473–508.

12. Lo GS, Goldberg AP, Lim A, Grundhauser JJ, Anderson C, Schonfeld G. Soy fiber improves lipid and carbohydrate metabolism in primary hyperlipidemic subjects. *Atherosclerosis.* 1986;62:239–248.

13. Topping DL. Soluble fiber polysaccharides: effects on plasma cholesterol and colonic fermentation. *Nutr Rev.* 1991;49:195–203.

14. Raper NR, Cronin FJ, Exler J. Omega-3 fatty acid content of the US food supply. *J Am Coll Nutr.* 1992;11:304–308.

15. Cunnane SC, Chen Z-Y, Yang J, Liede AC, Hammadeh M, Crawford MA. Alpha-linolenic acid in humans: direct functional role or dietary precursor? *Nutrition.* 1991;7:437–439.

16. Winter R. *Super Soy: The Miracle Bean.* New York: Crown Trade Paperbacks; 1996.

17. Kudchodkar BJ, Horlick L, Sodhi HS. Effects of plant sterols on cholesterol metabolism in man. *Atherosclerosis.* 1976;23: 239–248.

18. Long WH, Jones PJ. Dietary phytosterols: a review of metabolism, benefits, and side effects. *Life Science.* 1995;57: 195–206.

19. Miettinen TA, Puska P, Gylling H, Vanhanen H, Vartiainen E. Reduction of serum cholesterol with sitostanol-ester margarine in a mildly hypercholesterolemic population. *N Engl J Med.* 1995;333:1308–1312.

20. Knuiman JT, Beynen AC, Katan MB. Lecithin intake and serum cholesterol. *Am J Clin Nutr.* 1980;49:266–268.

21. Blusztajn JK. Choline, a vital amine. *Science.* 1998;281: 794–795.

22. Seibel MM. The role of nutrition and nutritional supplements in women's health. *Fertil Steril.* 1999;72:579–591.

23. Lindsay DR, Kelly RW. The metabolism of phyto-estrogens in sheep. *Austr Vet J.* 1970;46:219–222.

24. Messina M, Messina V, Setchell K. *The Simple Soybean and Your Health.* Garden City Park, NY: Avery Publishing Group; 1994.

25. Adlercreutz H, Mazur W. Phyto-estrogens and western diseases. *Ann Int Med.* 1997;29:95–120.

26. Persky VW, Turyk ME, Wang L, et al. Effect of soy protein on endogenous hormones in postmenopausal women. *Am J Clin Nutr.* 2002; 75:145–153.

CHAPTER 4

1. Sheehy G. *The Silent Passage.* New York: Pocket Books; 1991.

2. Haines CJ, Chung TKH, Leung DHY. A prospective study of

the frequency of acute menopausal symptoms in Hong Kong Chinese women. *Maturitas.* 1994;18:175–181.

3. Adlercreutz H, Hamalainen E, Gorbach S, Goldin B. Dietary phyto-oestrogens and the menopause in Japan. *Lancet.* 1992;339:1233.

4. Murkies AL, Lombard C, Strauss BJG, Wilcox G, Burger HG, Morton MS. Dietary flour supplementation decreases postmenopausal hot flushes: effect of soy and wheat. *Maturitas.* 1995;21:189–195.

5. Brzezinski A, Adlercreutz H, Shaoul R, et al. Short-term effects of phytoestrogen-rich diet on postmenopausal women. *Menopause.* 1997;4:89–94.

6. Albertazzi P, Pansini F, Bonaccorsi G, Zanotti L, Forini E, De Aloysio D. The effect of dietary soy supplementation on hot flushes. *Obstet Gynecol.* 1998;91:6–11.

7. Somekawa Y, Chiguchi M, Ishibashi T, Takeshi A. Soy intake related to menopausal symptoms, serum lipids, and bone mineral density in postmenopausal Japanese women. *Obstet Gynecol.* 2001;97:109–115.

8. Scambia G, Mango D, Signorile PG, et al. Clinical effects of a standardized soy extract in postmenopausal women: a pilot study. *Menopause.* 2000;7:105–111.

9. Upmalis DH, Lobo R, Bradley L, Warren M, Cone FL, Lamia CA. Vasomotor symptom relief by soy isoflavone extract tablets in postmenopausal women: a multicenter, double-blind, randomized, placebo-controlled study. *Menopause.* 2000;7:236–242.

10. Haas S, Walsh B, Evans S, et al. The effect of transdermal estradiol on hormone and metabolic dynamics over a six-week period. *Obstet Gynecol.* 1988;71:671–676.

11. Shaver JLF, Giblin E, Pauslen V. Sleep quality subtypes in midlife women. *Sleep.* 1991;14:18–23.

12. Birnholtz JC. Sexual lubricants: promoting health and pleasure. *Human Sexuality.* April 1998;1:19–24.

13. Wilcox G, Wahlqvist ML, Burger HG, Medley G. Oestrogenic effects of plant foods in postmenopausal women. *BMJ*. 1990;301:905–909.

CHAPTER 5

1. Cummings SR, Black DM, Rubin SM. Lifetime risks of hip, Colles', or vertebral fracture and coronary heart disease among white postmenopausal women. *Arch Intern Med*. 1989;149:2445–2448.

2. Epstein S, Goodman GR. Improved strategies for diagnosis and treatment of osteoporosis. *Menopause*. 1999;6:242–250.

3. Riggs BL. Overview of osteoporosis. *West J Med*. Jan 1991;154:63–77.

4. Ray NF, Chan JK, Thamer M, Melton LJ III. Medical expenditures for the treatment of osteoporotic fractures in the United States in 1995. *Report from the National Osteoporosis Foundation*. 1997;12:24–35.

5. Minkin MJ, Wright CV. *What Every Woman Needs to Know About Menopause*. New Haven, Conn.: Yale University Press; 1996:55.

6. National Osteoporosis Foundation. Physicians guide to prevention and treatment of osteoporosis. *Excerpta Medica*. 1998.

7. McClung MR. Clinical utility of bone density testing. *Menopause Management*. 2000;9:6–12.

8. Hodgson CR, Johnston CC Jr. AACE clinical practice guidelines for the prevention and treatment of postmenopausal osteoporosis. *Endocr Pract*. 1996;2:157–171.

9. Clarke BL. Does knowledge of bone density improve evaluation and management of postmenopausal osteoporosis? *Endocr Pract*. 2000;6:407–409.

10. Schneider DL, Barrett-Connor EL. Urinary N-telopeptide levels discriminate normal, osteopenic, and osteoporotic bone mineral density. *Arch Intern Med*.1997;157:1241–1245.

11. Finn SC. The skeleton crew: is calcium enough? *J Womens Health.* 1998;7:31–36.

12. Seibel MM. The role of nutrition and nutritional supplements in women's health. *Fertil Steril.* 1999;72:579–591.

13. Tylarksy FA, Bortz AD, Hancock RL, Anderson JJ. Familial resemblance of radial bone mass between premenopausal mothers and their college-age daughters. *Calcif Tissue Int.* 1989;45:265–271.

14. Chapuy MC, Arlot ME, Duboeuf F, et al. Vitamin D_3 and calcium to prevent hip fractures in elderly women. *N Engl J Med.* 1992;327:1637–1642.

15. Packard PT, Heaney RP. Medical nutrition therapy for patients with osteoporosis. *J Am Diet Assoc.* 1997;97:414–418.

16. Ibid.

17. Dawson-Hughes B. Osteoporosis treatment and the calcium requirement. *Am J Clin Nutr.* 1998;67:5–6.

18. Heaney RP, et al. Influence of calcium load on absorption fraction. *J Bone Min Res.* 1990;5:1135–1138.

19. Dawson-Hughes B. Calcium and osteoporosis. *Alternative therapies in women's health. American Health Consultants.* 2000;2(4):25–32.

20. Arjmandi BH, Birnbaum R, Noopur VG, et al. Bone-sparing effect of soy protein in ovarian hormone-deficient rats is related to its isoflavone content. *Am J Clin Nutr.* 1998;68 (suppl):1364S-1368S.

21. Heaney RP, Weaver CM. Effect of psyllium on absorption of coingested calcium. *J Am Geriatr Soc.* 1995;43:261–263.

22. Heaney RP. Nutritional factors in osteoporosis. *Ann Rev Nutr.* 1993;13:287–316.

23. Levenson DI, Ohayon KA. A practical analysis of calcium supplements. *Alternative therapies in women's health. American Health Consultants.* 2000;2(4):28–32.

24. Levenson DE, Bockman RS. A review of calcium preparations. *Nutr Rev.* 1994;52:221–232.

25. Whiting SJ. Safety of some calcium supplements questioned. *Nutr Rev.* 1994;52:95–97.

26. Rahwan RG. Cancer therapies: approved, unapproved, and experimental. *US Pharmacist.* 2000;25:HS-3–26.

27. Wortsman J, Matsuoka LY, Tai CC, Lu Z, Holick MF. Decreased bioavailability of vitamin D in obesity. *Am J Clin Nutr.* 2000;72:690–693.

28. Wester P. Magnesium. *Am J Clin Nutr.* 1987;45:1305–1312.

29. Franz KB. Magnesium intake during pregnancy. *Magnesium.* 1987;6:18–27.

30. Fugh-Berman A. Dietary supplements for migraine: magnesium and riboflavin. *Alternative therapies in women's health. American Health Consultants.* 1999;1(3):17–19.

31. Lewis LL, Shaver JF, Woods NF, et al. Bone resorption levels by age and menopausal status in 5,157 women. *Menopause.* 2000;7:42–52.

32. Michaelsson K, Baron JA, Farahmand BY, et al. Hormone replacement therapy and risk of hip fracture: population based case-control study. *BMJ.* 1998;316:1858–1863.

33. Arjmandi BH, Alekel L, Hollis BW, et al. Dietary soybean protein prevents bone loss in an ovariectomized rat model of osteoporosis. *J Nutr.* 1996;126:161–167.

34. Arjmandi BH, Birnbaum R, Goyal NV, et al. Bone-sparing effect of soy protein in ovarian hormone-deficient rats is related to its isoflavone content. *Am J Clin Nutr.* 1998;68(suppl): 1364S–1368S.

35. Anderson JJ, Ambrose WW, Garner SC. Biphasic effects of genistein on bone tissue in the ovariectomized, lactating rat model. *Proc Soc Exp Biol Med.* 1998;217:345–350.

36. Blair HC, Jordan E, Peterson TG, Barnes S. Variable effects of tyrosine kinase inhibitors on avian osteoclastic activity and reduction of bone loss in ovariectomized rats. *J Cell Biochem.* 1996;61:629–637.

37. Ishida H, Uesugi T, Hirai K, et al. Preventive effects of the

plant isoflavones, daidzin and genistin, on bone loss in ovariectomized rats fed a calcium-deficient diet. *Biol Pharm Bull.* 1998;21:62–66.

38. Yamaguchi M, Gao YH. Anabolic effect of genistein and genistin on bone metabolism in the femoral-metaphyseal tissues of elderly rats: the genistein effect is enhanced by zinc. *Mol Cell Biochem.* 1998;178:377–382.

39. Adlercreutz H, Mazur W. Phyto-oestrogens and western diseases. *Ann Int Med.* 1997;29:95–120.

40. Tsunenari T, Yamada S, Kawakatsu M, Negishi H, Tsutsumi M. Menopause-related changes in bone mineral density in Japanese women: a longitudinal study on lumbar spine and proximal femur. *Calcif Tissue Int.* 1995;56:5–10.

41. Potter SM, Baum JA, Teng H, Stillman RJ, Shay NF, Erdman JW Jr. Soy protein and isoflavones: their effects on blood lipids and bone density in postmenopausal women. *Am J Clin Nutr.* 1998;68(6 suppl):1375S–1379S.

42. Alekel DL, St Germain A, Peterson CT, Hanson KB, Stewart JW, Toda T. Isoflavone-rich soy protein isolate attenuates bone loss in the lumbar spine of perimenopausal women. *Am J Clin Nutr.* 2000;72:844–852.

43. Murkies AL, Wilcox G, Davis SR. Phytoestrogens. *J Clin Endocrinol Metab.* 1998;83:297–303.

44. Gallagher JC, Rafferty K, Haynatzka V, Wilson M. The effect of soy protein on bone metabolism. *J Nutr.* 2000;130:667S.

45. Bonaccorsi G, Albertazzi P, Canstantino D, et al. Soy phytoestrogens and bone. N Am Menopause Soc Meet. 1997;44.

46. Cecchini MG, Fleisch H, Muhlbauer RC. Ipriflavone inhibits bone resorption in intact and ovariectomized rats. *Calcif Tissue Int.* 1997;61:S9–S11.

47. Notoya K, Yoshida K, Tsukuda R, Taketomi S, Tsuda M. Increase in femoral bone mass by ipriflavone alone and in combination with alpha-hydroxy vitamin D_3 in growing rats with skeletal unloading. *Calcif Tissue Int.* 1996;58:88–94.

48. Ghezzo C, Civitelli R, Cadel S, et al. Ipriflavone does not alter bone apatite crystal structure in adult male rats. *Calcif Tissue Int.* 1996;59:496–499.

49. Scheiber MD, Rebar RW. Isoflavones and postmenopausal bone health: a viable alternative to estrogen therapy? *Menopause.* 1999;6:233–241.

50. Gambacciani M, Cappagli B, Paggesi L, Ciaponi M, Genazzani AR. Ipriflavone prevents the loss of bone mass in pharmacological menopause induced by GnRH-agonists. *Calcif Tissue Int.* 1997;61:S15–S18.

51. Gambacciani M, Spinetti A, Cappagli B, et al. Effects of ipriflavone administration on bone mass and metabolism in ovariectomized women. *J Endocrinol Invest.* 1993;16:333–337.

52. Gennari C, Agnusdei D, Crepaldi G, et al. Effects of ipriflavone—a synthetic derivative of natural isoflavones on bone mass and loss in the early years after menopause. *Menopause.* 1998;5:9–15.

53. Melis GB, Paoletti AM, Cagnacci A. Ipriflavone prevents bone loss in postmenopausal women. *Menopause.* 1996; 3:27–32.

54. Gennari C, Adami S, Agnusdei D, et al. Effect of chronic treatment with ipriflavone in postmenopausal women with low bone mass. *Calcif Tissue Int.* 1997;61:S19–S22.

55. Ushiroyama T, Okamura S, Ikeda A, Ueki M. Efficacy of ipriflavone and 1-alpha vitamin D therapy for the cessation of vertebral bone loss. *Int J Gynaecol Obstet.* 1995;48:283–288.

56. Brandi ML. Ipriflavone: new insights into its mechanism of action on bone remodeling. *Calcif Tissue Int.* 1993;52:151–152.

CHAPTER 6

1. Anthony MS, Clarkson TB, Williams JK. Effects of soy isoflavones on atherosclerosis: potential mechanisms. *Am J Clin Nutr.* 1998;68(suppl):1390S–1393S.

2. *Health Care Financing Review.* Statistical Supplement. HCFA; 1999.

3. American Heart Association. 2001 heart and stroke statistical update. Dallas: American Heart Association; 2000.

4. Rich-Edwards JW, Manson JE, Hennekens CH, Buring JE. The primary prevention of coronary heart disease in women. *N Engl J Med.* 1995;332:1758–1765.

5. Murabito JM. Women and cardiovascular disease. Contributions from the Framingham Heart Study. *J Am Med Wom Assoc.* 1995;50:35–39.

6. Strong WB, Dennison BA. Pediatric preventive cardiology: atherosclerosis and coronary heart disease. *Pediatric Review.* 1988;9:303–314.

7. American Heart Association. 1997 Heart and stroke statistical update. Dallas: American Heart Association; 1996. AHA publication 55-0524.

8. Online Heart & Stroke A–Z Guide. American Heart Association, 2001: *www.americanheart.org*

9. Enos WF, Holmes RH, Beyer J. Coronary disease among United States soldiers killed in action in Korea. *JAMA.* 1953;152:1090–1093.

10. Ornish D, Brown SE, Scherwitz LW, et al. Can lifestyle changes reverse coronary heart disease? *Lancet.* 1990; 336:129.

11. Wenger NK. Hypertension and other cardiovascular risk factors in women. *Am J Hypertens.* 1995;8:94S–99S.

12. Manson JE, Colditz GA, Stampfer MJ, et al. A prospective study of obesity and risk of coronary heart disease in women. *N Engl J Med.* 1990;322:882–889.

13. Willet WC, Manson JE, Stampfer MJ, et al. Weight, weight change, and coronary heart disease in women. Risk within the "normal" weight range. *JAMA.* 1995;273:461–465.

14. Flavell CM. Women and coronary heart disease. *Prog Cardiovasc Nurs.* 1994;9:18–27.

15. American Diabetes Association. *Diabetes Facts. Women and Diabetes*. Alexandria, Va: American Diabetes Association; 1998.

16. National Health and Nutrition Examination Survey (1988–1994). *Heart and Stroke Guide*. American Heart Association, 2001: *www.americanheart.org*.

17. Rich-Edwards JW, Manson JE, Hennekens CH, Buring JE. The primary prevention of coronary heart disease in women. *N Engl J Med*. 1995;332:1758–1765.

18. Federation of American Societies for Experimental Biology, Life Sciences Research Office. Prepared for the interagency Board for Nutrition Monitoring and Related Research. Third Report on Nutrition Monitoring in the United States. Washington, DC: U.S. Government Printing Office; 1995.

19. Hoerger TJ, Bala MV, Bray JW, et al. Treatment patterns and distribution of low density lipoprotein cholesterol levels in treatment-eligible United States adults. *Am J Cardiol*. 1998;82:61–65.

20. O'Brien T, Nguyen TT. Lipids and lipoproteins in women. *Mayo Clin Proc*. 1997;72:235–244.

21. Spady KD, Dietschy JM. Interaction of dietary cholesterol and triglycerides in the regulation of hepatic low density lipoprotein transport in the hamster. *J Clin Invest*. 1988; 81:300–309.

22. Simopoulos AT. Trans fatty acids. In: Spiller GE, ed. *Handbook of Lipids in Human Nutrition*. Boca Raton, Fla: CRC Press; 1996:96.

23. Willet WC, Stampfer MJ, Manson JE, et al. Intake of trans fatty acids and risk of coronary heart disease among women. *Lancet*. 1993;341:581–585.

24. Physician advice and individual behaviors about cardiovascular disease risk reduction—seven states and Puerto Rico, 1997. *MMWR*. 1999;48:74–77.

25. Somekawa Y, Chiguchi M, Ishibashi T, Aso T. Soy intake re-

lated to menopausal symptoms, serum lipids, and bone mineral density in postmenopausal Japanese women. *Obstet Gynecol.* 2001;97:109–115.

26. Chen J, Gao J. The Chinese total diet study in 1990: part II. Nutrients. *J AOAC Int.* 1993;76:1206–1211.

27. Ornish D, Scherwitz LW, Billings JH, et al. Intensive lifestyle changes for reversal of coronary heart disease. *JAMA.* 1998;380:2001–2007.

28. Hodges RE, Krehl WA, Stoné DB, Lopez A. Dietary carbohydrates and low cholesterol diets: effects on serum lipids of man. *Am J Clin Nutr.* 1967;20:198.

29. Sirtori CR, Agradi E, Conti F, Mantero O, Gatti E. Soybean-protein diet in the treatment of type-II hyperlipoproteinaemia. *Lancet.* 1977;5:275–277.

30. Anderson JW, Johnstone BM, Cook-Newell ME. Meta-analysis of the effects of soy protein intake on serum lipids. *N Engl J Med.* 1995;333:276–282.

31. Cassidy A, Bingham S, Setchell KD. Biological effects of soy protein rich in isoflavones on the menstrual cycle of premenopausal women. *Am J Clin Nutr.* 1994;60:333–340.

32. Meinertz H, Nilausen K, Faergeman O. Soy protein and casein in cholesterol-enriched diets: effects on plasma lipoproteins in normolipidemic subjects. *Am J Clin Nutr.* 1989;50: 786–793.

33. Wangen KE, Duncan AM, Xu X, Kurzer MS. Soy isoflavones improve plasma lipids in normocholesterolemic and mildly hypercholesterolemic postmenopausal women. *Am J Clin Nutr.* 2001;73:225–231.

34. Gardner CD, Newell KA, Cherin R, Haskell WL. The effect of soy protein with or without isoflavones relative to milk protein on plasma lipids in hypercholesterolemic postmenopausal women. *Am J Clin Nutr.* 2001;73:728–735.

35. Nestel PJ, Yamashita T, Sasahara T, et al. Soy isoflavones improve systemic arterial compliance but not plasma lipids in

menopausal and perimenopausal women. *Arterioscler Thromb Vasc Biol.* 1997;17:3392–3398.

36. Sirtori CR, Lovati MR, Manzoni C, Monetti M, Pazzucconi F, Gatti E. Soy and cholesterol reduction: clinical experience. *J Nutr.* 1995;125:598S–605S.

37. Tham DM, Gardner CD, Haskell WL. Potential health benefits of dietary phytoestrogens: a review of the clinical, epidemiological, and mechanistic evidence. *J Clin Endocrinol Metab.* 1998;83:2223–2235.

38. Topping DL. Soluble fiber polysaccharides: effects on plasma cholesterol and colonic fermentation. *Nutr Rev.* 1991;49: 195–203.

39. Messina M, Messina V, Setchell K. *The Simple Soybean and Your Health.* Garden City Park, NY: Avery Publishing Group; 1994.

40. Sanchez A, Hubbard RW. Plasma amino acids and the insulin/glucagon ratio as an explanation for the dietary protein modulation of atherosclerosis. *Med Hypoth.* 1991;35:324–329.

41. Fang Z, Chen YF, Oparil S, Wyss JM. Induction of dietary NaCl-sensitive hypertension in female spontaneously hypertensive rats: role of estrogen. *Hypertension.* 1999;34:336. Abstract.

42. Hodgson JM, Puddey IB, Beilin IJ, et al. Effects of isoflavonoids on blood pressure in subjects with high-normal ambulatory blood pressure levels: a randomized controlled trial. *Am J Hypertens.* 1999;12:47–53.

43. Washburn S, Burke GL, Morgan T, Anthony M. Effect of soy protein supplementation on serum lipoproteins, blood pressure, and menopausal symptoms in perimenopausal women. *Menopause.* 1999;6:7–13.

44. Anthony MS, Clarkson TB. Comparison of soy phytoestrogens and conjugated equine estrogens on atherosclerosis progression in postmenopausal monkeys. *Circulation.* 1998;97:829. Abstract.

45. Williams JK, Honore EK, Washburn SA, Clarkson TB. Effects of hormone replacement therapy on reactivity of atherosclerotic coronary arteries in cynomolgus monkeys. *J Am Coll Cardiol.* 1994;24:1757–1761.

46. Tikkanen MJ, Wahala K, Ojala S, Vihma V, Adlercreutz H. Effect of soybean phytoestrogen intake on low density lipoprotein oxidation resistance. *Proc Natl Acad Sci USA.* 1998;95:3106–3110.

47. Nestel PJ, Yamashita T, Sasahara T, et al. Soy isoflavones improve systemic arterial compliance but not plasma lipids in menopausal and perimenopausal women. *Arterioscler Thromb Vasc Biol.* 1997;17:3392–3398.

48. McGrath BP, Liang YL, Teede H, Shiel LM, Cameron JD, Dart A. Age-related deterioration in arterial structure and function in postmenopausal women: impact of hormone replacement therapy. *Arterioscler Thromb Vasc Biol.* 1998; 18:1149–1156.

49. Honore EK, Williams JK, Anthony MS, Clarkson TB. Soy isoflavones enhance coronary vascular reactivity in atherosclerotic female macaques. *Fertil Steril.* 1997;67:148–164.

50. Anthony MS, Clarkson TB. Comparison of soy phytoestrogens and conjugated equine estrogens on atherosclerosis progression in postmenopausal monkeys. *Circulation.* 1998; 97:829. Abstract.

51. Kapiotis S, Hermann M, Held I, Seelos C, Ehringer H, Gmeiner BM. Genistein, the dietary-derived angiogenesis inhibitor, prevents LDL oxidation and protects endothelial cells from damage by atherogenic LDL. *Arterioscler Thromb Vasc Biol.* 1997;17:2868–2874.

52. Clarkson TB. Soy phytoestrogens: what will be their role in postmenopausal hormone replacement therapy? *Menopause.* 2000;7:71–75.

53. Verrillo A, de Teresa A, Giarrusso PC, La Rocca S. Soybean

protein diets in the management of type II hyperlipoproteinaemia. *Atherosclerosis.* 1985;54:321–331.

CHAPTER 7

1. American Institute for Cancer Research. *Diet and Health Recommendations for Cancer Prevention.* Washington, DC: 1998.

2. Cooper GM. *The Cancer Book.* Sudbury, Mass: Jones and Bartlett Publishers; 1993.

3. Shields PG, Harris CC. Molecular epidemiology and the genetics of environmental cancer. *JAMA.* 1991;266:681–687.

4. Cohen SM, Ellwein LB. Genetic factors, cell proliferation, and carcinogenesis. *Cancer Res.* 1991;51:6493–6505.

5. Cooper GM. *Oneogenes.* Sudbury, Mass: Jones and Bartlett Publishers; 1990.

6. Adlercreutz H. Phytoestrogens: epidemiology and a possible role in cancer protection. *Environ Health Perspect.* 1995; 103(suppl 7):103–112.

7. Akiyama T, Ishida J, Nakagawa S, et al. Genistein: a specific inhibitor of tyrosine-specific protein kinase. *J Biol Chem.* 1987;262:5592–5595.

8. Shivapurkar N, Tang Z, Alabaster O. The effect of high-risk and low-risk diets on aberrant crypt and colonic tumor formation in Fischer-344 rats. *Carcinogenesis.* 1992;13:887–890.

9. Yanagihara K, Ito A, Toge T, Numoto M. Antiproliferative effects of isoflavones on human cancer cell lines established from the gastrointestinal tract. *Cancer Res.* 1993;53: 5815–5821.

10. Fotsis T, Pepper M, Adlercreutz H, et al. Genistein, a dietary-derived inhibitor of in vitro angiogenesis. *Proc Natl Acad Sci USA.* 1993;90:2990–2994.

11. Kennedy AR. In vitro studies of anticarcinogenic protease in-

hibitors. In: Troll W, Kennedy AR, eds. *Protease Inhibitors as Cancer Chemopreventive Agents*. New York: Plenum Press; 1993:65–91.

12. Kennedy AR. The Bowman-Birk inhibitor from soybeans as an anticarcinogenic agent. *Am J Clin Nutr*. 1998;68(suppl): 1406S–1412S.

13. Kennedy AR. Prevention of carcinogenesis by protease inhibitors. *Cancer Res*. 1994;54(suppl):1999S–2005S.

14. Kudchodkar BJ, Horlick L, Sodhi HS. Effects of plant sterols on cholesterol metabolism in man. *Atherosclerosis*. 1976; 23:239–248.

15. Long WH, Jones PJ. Dietary phytosterols: a review of metabolism, benefits, and side effects. *Life Science*. 1995;57: 195–206.

16. Yoshiki Y, Kahara T, Iida T, Okubo K, Kanazawa T. Chemical structure and radical scavenging activity of soybean glycosides. *Am J Clin Nutr*. 1998;68:1528S.

17. Barber DA, Harris SR. Oxygen free radicals and antioxidants: a review. *American Pharmacy*. 1994;34:26–35.

18. Rao AV. Anticarcinogenic properties of plant saponins. *Am J Clin Nutr*. 1998;68:1528S.

19. Thompson LU, Zhang L. Phytic acid and minerals: effect on early markers of risk for mammary and colon carcinogenesis. *Carcinogenesis*. 1991;12:2041–2045.

20. Graf E, Eaton JW. Suppression of colonic cancer by dietary phytic acid. *Nutr Cancer*. 1993;19:11–19.

21. Beard JL. Are we at risk for heart disease because of normal iron status? *Nutr Rev*. 1993;51:112–115.

22. Wang HJ, Murphy P. Isoflavone content in commercial soybean foods. *J Agric Food Chem*. 1994;42;1666–1673.

23. Akiyama T, Ishida J, Nakagawa S, et al. Genistein, a specific inhibitor of tyrosine-specific protein kinases. *J Biol Chem*. 1987;262:5592–5595.

24. Fotsis T, Pepper M, Adlercreutz H, et al. Genistein, a derived

inhibitor of in vitro angiogenesis. *Proc Natl Acad Sci USA.* 1993;90:2690–2694.

25. Okura A, Arakawa H, Oka H, Yoshinari T, Monden Y. Effects of genistein on topoisomerase activity and on the growth of [Val 12]Ha-ras-transformed NIH 3T3 cells. *Biochem Biophys Res Commun.* 1988;157:183–189.

26. Watanabe T, Kondo K, Oishi M. Induction of in-vitro differentiation of mouse erythroleukemia cells by genistein, and inhibitor of tyrosine kinases. *Cancer Res.* 1991;51:764–768.

27. Constantinou A, Huberman E. Genistein as an inducer of tumor cell differentiation: possible mechanisms of action (43841). *Proc Soc Exp Biol Med.* 1995;208:109–115.

28. Gyorgy P, Murata K, Ikehata H. Antioxidants isolated from fermented soybeans (tempeh). *Nature.* 1963;204: 870–872.

29. Wei H, Bowen R, Cai Q, Barnes S, Wang Y. Antioxidant and antipromotional effects of the soybean isoflavone genistein. *Proc Soc Exp Biol Med.* 1995;208:124–130.

30. Adlercreutz H, Mousavi Y, Hockerstedt K. Diet and breast cancer. *Acta Oncol.* 1992;31:175–181.

31. Adlercreutz H, Honjo H, Higashi A, et al. Urinary excretion of lignans and isoflavonoid phytoestrogens in Japanese men and women consuming a traditional Japanese diet. *Am J Clin Nutr.* 1991;54:1093–1100.

32. Lee HP, Gourley L, Duffy SW, Esteve J, Lee J, Day NE. Dietary effects on breast-cancer risk in Singapore. *Lancet.* 1991;337:1197–1200.

33. Zheng W, Dai Q, Custer LJ, et al. Urinary excretion of isoflavonoids and the risk of breast cancer. *Cancer Epidemiol Biomarkers Prev.* 1999;8(1):35–40.

34. Wu AH, Ziegler RG, Horn-Ross PL, et al. Tofu and risk of breast cancer in Asian-Americans. *Cancer Epidemiol Biomarkers Prev.* 1996;5:901–906.

35. Murkies A, Dalais FS, Briganti EM, et al. Phytoestrogens and

breast cancer in postmenopausal women: a case control study. *Menopause.* 2000;7:289–296.

36. Barnes S, Grubbs C, Setchell KDR, Carlson J. Soybeans inhibit mammary tumors in models of breast cancer. In: Pariza M., ed. *Mutagens and Carcinogens in the Diet.* New York: Wiley-Liss, Inc.; 1990:239–253.

37. Barnes S, Peterson TG, Grubbs C, Setchell KDR. Potential role of dietary isoflavones in the prevention of cancer. In: Jacobs MM, ed. *Diet and Cancer: Markers.* New York: John Wiley & Sons; 1994.

38. Xu X, Rossi H, Pezzuto JM, et al. Soy protein isolate depleted of isoflavones prevents DMBA-induced mammary tumors in female rats. March 2000. Proceedings of the American Association for Cancer Research Annual Meeting. Champaign, Ill: University of Illinois; April 1–5, 2000.

39. Constantinou AI, Krygier AE, Mehta RR. Genistein induces maturation of cultured human breast cancer cells and prevents tumor growth in nude mice. *Am J Clin Nutr.* 1998;68(suppl):1426S-1430S.

40. Peterson G, Barnes S. Genistein inhibition of the growth of human breast cancer cells—independence from estrogen receptors and the multi-drug resistance gene. *Biochem Biophys Res Commun.* 1991;179:661–667.

41. Hoffman R. Potent inhibition of breast cancer cell lines by the isoflavonoid kievitone: comparison with genistein. *Biochem Biophys Res Commun.* 1995;211:600–606.

42. Monti E, Sinha BK. Antiproliferative effect of genistein and adriamycin against estrogen-dependent and -independent human breast carcinoma cell lines. *Anticancer Res.* 1994;14:1221–1226.

43. Verma SP, Goldin BR. Effect of soy-derived isoflavonoids on the induced growth of MCF-7 cells by estrogenic environmental chemicals. *Nutr Cancer.* 1998;30(3):232–239.

44. Lu LJ, Anderson KE, Grady JJ, Kohen F, Nagamani M. De-

creased ovarian hormones during a soya diet: implications for breast cancer prevention. *Cancer Res.* 2000;60:4112–4121.

45. Lu LJ, Cree M, Josyula S, Nagamani M, Grady JJ, Anderson KE. Increased urinary excretion of 2-hydroxyestrone but not 16-alpha-hydroxyestrone in premenopausal women during a soya diet containing isoflavones. *Cancer Res.* 2000; 60: 1299–1305.

46. Russo J, Russo IH. DNA labeling index and structure of the rat mammary gland as determinants of its susceptibility to carcinogenesis. *JNCI.* 1978;61:1451–1459.

47. Russo IH, Koszalka M, Russo J. Effect of human chorionic gonadotrophins on mammary gland differentiation and carcinogenesis. *Carcinogenesis.* 1990;11:1849–1855.

48. White E, Velentgas P, Mandelson MT, et al. Variation in mammographic density by the time in menstrual cycle among women aged 40–49 years. *JNCI.* 1998;90:906–910.

49. Lamartiniere CA, Zhang J-X, Cotroneo MS. Genistein studies in rats: potential for breast cancer prevention and reproductive and developmental toxicity. *Am J Clin Nutr.* 1998;68(suppl):1400S–1405S.

50. Quak SH, Tan SP. Use of soy-protein formulas and soyfood for feeding infants and children in Asia. *Am J Clin Nutr.* 1998;68(suppl):1444S–1446S.

51. Setchell KDR, Zimmer-Nechemias L, Cai J, Heubi JE. Isoflavone content of infant formulas and the metabolic fate of these phytoestrogens in early life. *Am J Clin Nutr.* 1998;68(suppl):1453S–1461S.

52. Hsieh CY, Santell RC, Haslam SZ. Estrogenic effects of genistein on the growth of estrogen receptor-positive human breast cancer (MCF-7) cells in vitro and in vivo. *Cancer Res.* 1998;58:3833–3838.

53. Wang C, Kurzer MS. Effects of phytoestrogens on DNA synthesis in MCF-7 cells in the presence of estradiol or growth factors. *Nutr Cancer.* 1998;31:90–100.

54. Zava DT, Duwe G. Estrogenic and antiproliferative properties of genistein and other flavonoids in human breast cancer cells in vitro. *Nutr Cancer.* 1997;27:31–40.

55. McMichael-Phillips DF, Harding C, Morton M, et al. Effects of soy-protein supplementation on epithelial proliferation in the histologically normal human breast. *Am J Clin Nutr.* 1998;68(suppl):1431S–1436S.

56. Hargreaves DF, Potten CS, Harding C. Two-week dietary soy supplementation has an estrogenic effect on normal pre-menopausal breast. *J Clin Endocrinol Metab.* 1999;84: 4017–4024.

57. Williams G, Anderson E, Howell A, et al. Oral contraceptive (OCP) use increases proliferation and decreases oestrogen receptor content of epithelial cells in the normal human breast. *Int J Cancer.* 1991;48:206–210.

58. Potten CS, Watson RJ, Williams GT, et al. The effect of age and menstrual cycle upon proliferative activity of the normal human breast. *Br J Cancer.* 1988;58:163–170.

59. Vincent A, Fitzpatrick LA. Soy isoflavones: are they useful in menopause? *Mayo Clinic Proc.* Nov 2000;75(11):1174–1184.

60. Lu LW, Anderson KE, Grady JJ, Nagamani M. Effects of soya consumption for one month on steroid hormones in premeno-pausal women: implications for breast cancer risk reduction. *Cancer Epidemiol, Biomarkers & Prevention.* 1996;5:63–70.

61. Webb D. Important update: should you take isoflavones. *Prevention.* June 2001;69–70.

62. Beckmann MW, Jap D, Djahansouzi S, et al. Hormone re-placement therapy after treatment of breast cancer: effects on postmenopausal symptoms, bone mineral density and re-currence rates. *Oncology.* 2001;60(3):199–206.

63. Col NF, Hirota LK, Orr RK, Erban JK, Wong JB, Lau J. Hor-mone replacement therapy after breast cancer: a systematic review and quantitative assessment of risk. *J Clin Oncol.* 2001;19(8):2357–2363.

64. Marsden J. Hormone replacement therapy and breast cancer. *Maturitas.* 2000;34(suppl 2):S11–S24.

65. Seibel MM. Soy and the treatment of menopause. In: Genazzani AR and Petraglia F, eds. *Advances in Gynecological Endocrinology.* London: Parthenon Publishing; 2001.

66. Pan Y, Anthony M, Watson S. Soy phytoestrogens improve radial arm maze performance in ovariectomized retired breeder rats and do not attenuate benefits of 17-β estradiol treatment. *Menopause.* 2000;7:230–235.

67. Foth D, Cline JM. Effects of mammalian and plant estrogens on mammary glands and uteri of macaques. *Am J Clin Nutr.* 1998;68:1413S–1417S.

68. Scambia G, Mango K, Signorile PG, et al. Clinical effects of standardized soy extract in postmenopausal women: a pilot study. *Menopause.* 2000;7:105–111.

69. Baird DD, Umbach DM, Sansdell L, et al. Dietary intervention study to assess estrogenicity of dietary soy among postmenopausal women. *J Clin Endocrinol Metab.* 1995;80(5): 1685–1690.

70. Wilcox G, Wahlqvist MS, Burger HG, et al. Oestrogenic effects of plant foods in postmenopausal women. *Br J Med.* 1990;301:905–906.

71. Bal DG. Cancer statistics 2001: quo vadis or whither goest thou? *CA Cancer J Clin.* 2001;51:11–14.

72. Messina M, Persky V, Setchell K, Barnes S. Soy intake and cancer risk: a review of the in vitro and in vivo data. *Nutr Cancer.* 1994;21:113–131.

73. Watanabe S, Doessel S. Colon cancer: an approach from molecular epidemiology. *J Epidemiol.* 1993;3:47–61.

74. Stephan AM, Cummings JH. The microbial contribution to human faecal mass. *J Med Microbiol.* 1980;13:45–56.

75. Messina M, Messina V, Setchell K. *The Simple Soybean and Your Health.* Garden City Park, NY: Avery Publishing Group; 1994:84.

76. Rackis JJ, Honig DH, Sessa DJ, Steggerda FR. Flavor and flatulence factors in soybean protein products. *J Agr Food Chem.* 1970;18:977–982.

77. Rhee YK, Bae EA, Kim SY, Han MJ, Choi EC, Kim DH. Antitumor activity of bifidobacterium sp. isolated from a healthy Korean. *Arch Pharm Res.* 2000;23(5):482–487.

78. Park HY, Bae EA, Han MJ, Choi EC, Kim DH. Inhibitory effects of bifidobacterium spp. isolated from a healthy Korean on harmful enzymes of human intestinal microflora. *Arch Pharm Res.* 1998;21(1):54–61.

79. Koo M, Rao AV. Long-term effect of bifidobacteria and neosugar on precursor lesions of colonic cancer in CF1 mice. *Nutr Cancer.* 1991;16:249–257.

80. Hata Y, Yamamoto M, Nakajima K. Effects of soybean oligosaccharides on human digestive organs: estimation of fifty percent effective dose and maximum non-effective dose based on diarrhea. *J Clin Biochem Nutr.* 1991;10:135–144.

81. Kim YI, Baik HW, Fawaz K, et al. Effects of folate supplementation on two provisional molecular markers of colon cancer: a prospective, randomized trial. *Am J Gastroenterol.* 2001;96:184–195.

82. Kampman E, Slattery ML, Caan B, Potter JD. Calcium, vitamin D, sunshine exposure, dairy products and colon cancer risk (United States). *Cancer Causes Control.* 2000;11: 459–466.

83. Adlercreutz H, Mazur W. Phyto-oestrogens and western diseases. *Ann Int Med.* 1997;29:95–120.

84. Slattery ML, Potter JD, Curtin K, et al. Estrogens reduce and withdrawal of estrogens increase risk of microsatellite instability-positive colon cancer. *Cancer Res.* 2001;61:126–130.

85. Singh S, Langman MJS. Oestrogen and colonic epithelial cell growth. *Gut.* 1995;37:737–739.

86. Calle EE, Miracle-McMahill HL, Thun MJ, Heath CW. Estrogen replacement therapy and risk of fatal colon cancer in a

prospective cohort of postmenopausal women. *JNCI.* 1995;87:517–523.

87. Rutqvist LE, Hohansson H, Signomklao T, Johansson U, Fornander T, Wilking N. Adjuvant tomoxifen therapy for early stage breast cancer and secondary primary malignancies. *JNCI.* 1995;87:645–651.

88. Adlercreutz H, Fotsis T, Kurzer MS, Wahala K, Makela T, Hase T. Isotope dilution gas chromatographic mass spectrometric method for the determination of unconjugated lignans and isoflavonoids in human feces, with preliminary results in omnivorous and vegetarian women. *Anal Biochem.* 1995; 225:101–108.

89. Messina M, Bennink M. Soyfoods, isoflavones and risk of colonic cancer: a review of the in vitro and in vivo data. *Baillieres Clin Endocrinol Metab.* 1998;12:707–728.

90. Salti GI, Grewal S, Mehta RR, Das Gupta TK, Boddie AW Jr, Constantinou AI. Genistein induces apoptosis and topoisomerase II-mediated DNA breakage in colon cancer cells. *Eur J Cancer.* 2000;36:796–802.

91. Booth C, Hargreaves DF, Hadfield JA, McGown AT, Potten CS. Isoflavones inhibit intestinal epithelial cell proliferation and induce apoptosis in vitro. *Br J Cancer.* 1999;80: 1550–1557.

92. Greenlee RT, Murray T, Bolden S, et al. Cancer statistics, 2000. *CA Cancer J Clin.* 2000;50:7–33.

93. Watanabe M, Nakayama T, Shiraishi T, et al. Comparative studies of prostate cancer in Japan versus the United States: a review. *Urol Oncol.* 2000;5:274–283.

94. Breslow NE, Chan CW, Dhom G, et al. Latent carcinoma of prostate at autopsy in seven areas. *Int J Cancer.* 1977; 20:680–688.

95. Yatani R, Chigusa I, Akazaki K, Stemmerman GN, Welsh RA, Correa P. Geographic pathology of latent prostatic cancer. *Int J Cancer.* 1982;29:611–616.

96.   Wiseman H. The therapeutic potential of phytoestrogens. *Expert Opin Investig Drugs.* 2000;9:1829–1840.

97.   Peterson G, Barnes S. Genistein and biochanin-A inhibit the growth of human prostate cancer cells but not epidermal growth factor receptor tyrosine autophosphorylation. *Prostate.* 1993;22:335–345.

98.   Adlercreutz H, Makela S, Pylkkanen L, et al. Dietary phytoestrogens and prostate cancer. *Proc Am Assoc Cancer Res.* 1995;36:687. Extended abstract.

99.   Shen JC, Klein RD, Wei Q, et al. Low-dose genistein induces cyclin-dependent kinase inhibitors and G(1) cell-cycle arrest in human prostate cancer cells. *Mol Carcinog.* 2000;29:92–102.

100. Alhasan SA, Ensley JF, Sarkar FH. Genistein induced molecular changes in a squamous cell carcinoma of the head and neck cell line. *Int J Oncol.* 2000;16:333–338.

CHAPTER 8

1.   Messina M, Descheemaker K, Erdman JW Jr. *Am J Clin Nutr.* 1998;68(suppl):1329S.

2.   Conquering Diabetes. A report of the congressionally established diabetes research working group. NIH Publication No. 99-4398; 1999.

3.   CDC National Diabetes Fact Sheet, November 1, 1998.

4.   Von Mering J, Minkowski O. Diabetes mellitus nach pankreas extirpation. *Arch Exp Pathol Pharmacol Leipzig.* 1890;26:371.

5.   Steiner DF, Bell GI, Rubenstein AH, Chan SJ. Chemistry and biosynthesis of the islet hormones: insulin, islet amyloid polypeptide (amylin), glucagon, somatostatin, pancreatic polypeptide. In: DeGroot LJ, Jameson JL, eds. *Endocrinology.* 4th ed. Philadelphia: WB Saunders; 2001:667–696.

6.   Hazlett BE. Historical perspective: the discovery of insulin. In: Davidson JK, ed. *Clinical Diabetes Mellitus, Problem Ori-*

ented Approach. 2nd edition. New York: Thieme Medical Publishers, Inc.; 1991.

7. Aoyama T, Fukui K, Nakamori T, et al. Effect of soy and milk whey protein isolates and their hydrolysates on weight reduction in genetically obese mice. *Biosci Biotechnol Biochem.* 2000;64:2594–2600.

8. Vidon C, Boucher P, Cachefo A, Peroni O, Diraison F, Beylot M. Effects of isoenergetic high-carbohydrate compared with high-fat diets on human cholesterol synthesis and expression of key regulatory genes of cholesterol metabolism. *Am J Clin Nutr.* 2001;73:874–884.

9. Friedenwald J, Ruhrah J. The use of the soy bean as a food in diabetes. *Am J Med Sci.* 1910;140:793.

10. Jenkins DJ, Wolever TM, Taylor RH, et al. Glycemic index of foods: a physiological basis for carbohydrate exchange. *Am J Clin Nutr.* 1981;34:362–366.

11. Winter R. *Super Soy: The Miracle Bean.* New York: Crown Trade Paperbacks; 1996.

12. Lo GS. Physiological effects and physicochemical properties of soy cotyledon fiber. *Adv Exp Med Biol.* 1990;270:49–66.

13. D'Amico G, Gentile MG, Manna G, et al. Effect of vegetarian soy diet on hyperlipidaemia in nephritic syndrome. *Lancet.* 1992;339:1131–1134.

14. Gentile MG, Fellin G, Cofano F, et al. Treatment of proteinuric patients with a vegetarian soy diet and fish oil. *Clin Nephrol.* 1993;40:315–320.

15. Lemann J. Composition of the diet and calcium kidney stones. *N Engl J Med.* 1993;328:880–882.

16. Curhan GC, Willett WC, Rimm EB, Stampfer MJ. Prospective study of dietary calcium and other nutrients and the risk of symptomatic kidney stones. *N Engl J Med.* 1993;328:833–838.

17. Robertson WG, Peacock M, Marshall DH. Prevalence of urinary stone disease in vegetarians. *Eur Urol.* 1982;8:334–339.

18. Broughtan TA. Gallstones. *Curr Treatment Options Gastroenter.* 1999;2:154–161.

19. Tseng M, Everhart JE, Sandler RS. Dietary intake and gallbladder disease: a review. *Public Health Nutr.* 1999;2: 161–172.

20. Attili AF, Scafato E, Marchioli R, Marfisi RM, Festi D. Diet and gallstones in Italy: the cross-sectional MICOL results. *Hepatology.* 1998;27:1492–1498.

21. Ortega RM, Gernandez-Azuela M, Encinas-Sotillos A, Andres P, Lopez-Sobaler AM. Differences in diet and food habits between patients with gallstones and controls. *J Am Coll Nutr.* 1997;16:88–95.

22. Ozben T. Biliary lipid composition and gallstone formation in rabbits fed on soy protein, cholesterol, casein and modified casein. *Biochem J.* 1989;263:293–296.

23. Tomotake H, Shimaoka I, Kayashita J, Yokoyama F, Nakajoh M, Kato N. A buckwheat protein product suppresses gallstone formation and plasma cholesterol more strongly than soy protein isolate in hamsters. *J Nutr.* 2000;130:1670–1674.

24. Kritchevsky D, Klurfeld DM. Influence of vegetable protein on gallstone formation in hamsters. *Am J Clin Nutr.* 1979;32:2174–2176.

25. American Heart Association. 1997 Heart & Stroke Statistical Update. Dallas: American Heart Association; 1996; AHA publication 55-0524.

26. Online Heart & Stroke A–Z Guide. American Heart Association; 2001: *www.americanheart.org.*

27. Yamori Y, Horie R. Community-based prevention of stroke: nutritional improvement in Japan. *Health Rep.* 1994;6: 181–188.

28. Medkova IL, Mosiakina LI, Pavlova VE, Bugaev VA, Koryshev VI. Balanced vegetarian diet in combined rehabilitation of patients suffering from ischemic heart disease. *Klin Med (Mosk).* 1997;75:28–31.

29. Messina M, Messina V, Setchell K. *The Simple Soybean and Your Health*. Garden City Park, NY: Avery Publishing Group; 1994.

30. Fang Z, Chen YF, Oparil S, Wyss JM. Induction of dietary NaCl-sensitive hypertension in female spontaneously hypertensive rats: role of estrogen. *Hypertension*. 1999;34:336. Abstract.

31. Hodgson JM, Puddey IB, Beilin IJ, et al. Effects of isoflavonoids on blood pressure in subjects with high-normal ambulatory blood pressure levels: a randomized controlled trial. *Am J Hypertens*. 1999;12:47–53.

32. Washburn S, Burke GL, Morgan T, Anthony M. Effect of soy protein supplementation serum lipoproteins, blood pressure, and menopausal symptoms in perimenopausal women. *Menopause*. 1999;6:7–13.

33. Anthony MS, Clarkson TB. Comparison of soy phytoestrogens and conjugated equine estrogens on atherosclerosis progression in postmenopausal monkeys. *Circulation*. 1998; 97:829. Abstract.

34. Williams JK, Honore EK, Washburn SA, Clarkson TB. Effects of hormone replacement therapy on reactivity of atherosclerotic coronary arteries in cynomolgus monkeys. *J Am Coll Cardiol*. 1994;24:1757–1761.

35. Tikkanen MJ, Wahala K, Ojala S, Vihma V, Adlercreutz H. Effect of soybean phytoestrogen intake on low density lipoprotein oxidation resistance. *Proc Natl Acad Sci USA*. 1998;95:3106–3110.

36. Nestel PJ, Yamashita T, Sasahara T, et al. Soy isoflavones improve systemic arterial compliance but not plasma lipids in menopausal and perimenopausal women. *Arterioscler Thromb Vasc Biol*. 1997;17:3392–3398.

37. McGrath BP, Liang YL, Teede H, Shiel LM, Cameron JD, Dart A. Age-related deterioration in arterial structure and function in postmenopausal women: impact of hormone replacement therapy. *Arterioscler Thromb Vasc Biol*. 1998;18:1149–1156.

38. Patel YT, Minocha A. Lactose intolerance: diagnosis and management. *Compr Ther.* 2000;26:246–250.

39. Busineo L, Bruno G, Giampietro PG. Soy protein for the prevention and treatment of children with cow-milk allergy. *Am J Clin Nutr.* 1998;68(suppl):1447S–1452S.

40. Dragan I, Stroescu V, Stoian I, Georgescu E, Baloescu R. Studies regarding the efficiency of Supro isolated soy protein in Olympic athletes. *Rev Roum Physiol.* 1992;29:63–70.

CHAPTER 9

1. Richman A, Witkowski JP. Herbs by the numbers: Whole Foods' third annual natural herbal product sales survey. *Whole Foods.* October 1997;20.

2. FDC Reports. *The Tan Sheet.* Chevy Chase, Md; 1998:14.

3. Seibel MM. The role of nutrition and nutritional supplements in women's health. *Fertil Steril.* 1999;72:579–591.

4. Knapp HR. Drug-nutrient interactions in medical training. *J Am Coll Nutr.* 1995;14:114–115.

5. Uhland V. Supplementing a practice. *Natural Business LOHAS J.* May/June 2000;55–56.

6. Eisenberg DM, Kessler C, Foster C, Norlock FE, Calkins DR, Delbanco TL. Unconventional medicine in the United States: prevalence, costs, and patterns of use. *N Engl J Med.* 1993;328:246–252.

7. Israelsen LD, Blumenthal M. FDA issues final rules for structure/function claims for dietary supplements under DSHEA. *HerbalGram.* 2000;48:32–38.

8. Foreman J. St. John's wort: less than meets the eye. *Boston Globe.* January 10, 2000; C1.

9. Larkin M. Surgery patients at risk for herb-anesthesia interactions. *Lancet.* 1999;354:1362.

10. Macht DL, Cook HM. A pharmacological note on *Cimicifuga. J Amer Pharm Assoc.* 1992;21:324–330.

11. Jarry H, Harnischfeger G, Duker E. Studies on the endocrine efficacy of the constituents of *Cimicifuga racemosa*: 2. In vitro binding of constituents to estrogen receptors. *Planta Med.* 1985;51(4):316–319.

12. Bradley PR. Black cohosh. *British Herbal Compendium.* Bournemoth, Dorset, England: British Herbal Medicine Association; 1992;41:12–15.

13. Beuscher N. *Cimicifuga racemosa* L.—black cohosh. *HerbalGram.* Spring 1996;19–27.

14. Struck D, Tegtmeier M, Harnischfeger G. Flavones in extracts of *Cimicifuga racemosa. Planta Med.* 1997;63:289–290.

15. Schindler H. The constituents of medicinal plants and testing methods for botanical tinctures. *Arzneimittel-Forsch.* 1992;2:547–549.

16. Nesselhut T, Schellhase C, Deitrich R, Kuhn W. *Arch Gynecol Obstet.* 1993;254:817–818.

17. Leung AY, Foster S. *Encyclopedia of Common Natural Ingredients.* New York: John Wiley & Sons, Inc.; 1996:88–89.

18. Koch E. Hormonal effect of plants. *Hippokrates.* 1944:15; 22–23.

19. Foster S. Black cohosh: *Cimicifuga racemosa. HerbalGram.* Winter 1999;35–50.

20. Stolze H. An alternative to treat menopausal complaints. *Gynecology.* 1982;3:14–16.

21. Daiber W. Climacteric complaints: success without using hormones—a phytotherapeutic agent lessens hot flushes, sweating and insomnia. *Arztliche Praxis.* 1983;35(65):1946–1947.

22. Vorberg G. Therapy of climacteric complaints. *Zeitschrift fur Allgemeinmedizin.* 1984;60:626–629.

23. Warnecke G. Influence of a phytopharmaceutical on climacteric complaints. *Die Meizinische Welt.* 1985;36:871–874.

24. Stoll W. Phytopharmacon influences atrophic vaginal epithelium: double-blind study—*Cimicifuga* vs. estrogenic substances. *Therapeuticum.* 1987;1:23–31.

25. Petho G. Climacteric complaints are often helped with black cohosh. *Arztliche Praxis*. 1987;47:1551–1553.

26. Lehmann-Willenbrock E, Riedel HH. Clinical and endocrinological examinations concerning therapy of climacteric symptoms following hysterectomy with remaining ovaries. *Zentralblatt fur Gynakologie*. 1988;110(10):611–618.

27. Duker E-M, Kopanski L, Jarry H, Wuttke W. Effects of extracts from *Cimicifuga racemosa* on gonadotropin release in menopausal women and ovariectomized rats. *Planta Med*. 1991;57:420–424.

28. Beuscher N. *Cimicifuga racemosa* L. black cohosh. *Zeitschrift fur Phytotherapie*. 1995;16:301–310. Reprint in English, Clay A. Reichert R. *Quarterly Review of Natural Medicine*. Spring 1996;19–27.

29. Nesselhut T, Schellhas C, Deitrich R, Kuhn W. *Arch Gynecol and Obstet*. 1993;254:817–818.

30. Adlercreutz H, Mazur W. Phyto-oestrogens and western diseases. *Ann Med*. 1997;29:95–120.

31. Brzezinski A, Debi A. Phytoestrogens: the "natural" selective estrogen receptor modulators? *Eur J Obstet Gynecol Reprod Biol*. 1999;85:47–51.

32. Wuttke W, Gorkow C, Jarry J. Dopaminergic compounds in *Vitex agnus castus*. In: Loew D, Rietbrock N, eds. *Phytopharmaka in Forschung und Klinischer Anwendung*. Darmstadt: Steinkopff Verlag; 81–91.

33. Hirata JD, Swiers LM, Zell B, Small R, Ettinger B. Does dong quai have estrogenic effects in postmenopausal women? A double-blind, placebo-controlled trial. *Fertil Steril*. 1997;68:981–986.

34. Nemecz G. Evening primrose. *US Pharmacist*. November 1998;85–94.

35. Chenoy R, Hussain S, Tayob Y, O'Brien PMS, Moss MY, Morse PF. Effect of oral gamalenic acid from evening primrose oil on menopausal flushing. *Br Med J*. 1994;308:501–503.

36. Horrobin DF. GLA gammalinolenic acid: an intermediate in essential fatty acid metabolism with potential as an ethical pharmaceutical and as a food. *Rev Contemp Pharmacother.* 1990;1:1–45.

37. Barber RJ, Templeman C, Morton T, Delley GE, Weat L. Randomized placebo-controlled trial of an isoflavone supplement and menopausal symptoms in women. *Climacteric.* 1999;2:85–92.

38. Knight DC, Howes JB, Eden JA. The effect of Promensil, an isoflavone extract, on menopausal symptoms. *Climacteric.* 1999;2:79–84.

39. Nachtigall LB, LaGrega L, Lee WW, et al. The effects of isoflavones derived from red clover on vasomotor symptoms and endometrial thickness. 9th International Menopause Society World Congress on the Menopause, October 17–21, 1999.

40. Mitchell J, Rook A. *Botanical Dermatology—Plants and Plant Products Injurious to the Skin.* Vancouver: Greengrass; 1979.

41. Blatt MHG, Wiesbader H, Kupperman HS. Vitamin E and climacteric syndrome. *Arch Intern Med.* 1953;91:792–796.

42. Barton DL, Loprinze CL, Quella SK, et al. Prospective evaluation of vitamin E for hot flashes in breast cancer survivors. *J Clin Oncol.* 1998;16:495–500.

43. Central nervous system. In: Schulz V, Hansel R, Tyler VE. *Rational Phytotherapy.* 3rd ed. New York: Springer; 1998: 37–50.

44. Braquet P. The ginkgolides: potent platelet-activating factor antagonists isolated from *Ginkgo biloba* L.: chemistry, pharmacology, and clinical applications. *Drugs of the Future.* 1987;12:643–699.

45. Schmid M, Schmoll H, eds. *Ginkgo.* Stuttgart: Wissenschaftliche Verlagsgesellschaft mbH; 1994.

46. LeBars PL, Katz MM, Berman N, et al for the North American EGb Study Group. A placebo-controlled, double blind,

randomized trial of an extract of *Ginkgo biloba* for dementia. *JAMA.* 1997;278:1327–1332.

47. Rowin J, Lewis SL. Spontaneous bilateral subdural hematomas associated with chronic *Ginkgo biloba* ingestion. *Neurology.* 1996;46:1775–1776.

48. Mathews MK. Association of *Ginkgo biloba* with intracellular hemorrhage. *Neurology.* 1998;50:1933–1934.

49. Peters H, et al. Demonstration of the efficacy of gingko biloba extract EGb 761 on intermittent claudication. *VASA.* 1998;27:106–110.

50. Pittler MH, Ernest E. *Ginkgo biloba* extract for the treatment of intermittent claudication: a meta-analysis of randomized trials. *Am J Med.* 2000;108:276–281.

51. *Tufts University Health & Nutrition Letter.* June 2001; 19:6.

52. Sirtori CR, Pazzucconi F, Colombo L, Battistin P, Bondioli A, Descheemaeker K. Double-blind study of the addition of high-protein soya milk v. cows' milk to the diet of patients with severe hypercholesterolemia and resistance to or intolerance of statins. *Br J Nutr.* 1999;82:79–80.

CHAPTER 10

1. Wen P. An acquired taste. *Boston Globe.* August 25, 2001: A1.

2. Rohwedder C., Trofimov Y. Europeans are still mad for their beef. *Wall Street Journal.* May 17, 2001.

3. Messina M, Messina V, Setchell K. *The Simple Soybean and Your Health.* Garden City Park, NY: Avery Publishing Group; 1994.

4. Winter R. *Super Soy: The Miracle Bean.* New York: Crown Trade Paperbacks; 1996.

5. Rombauer IS, Becker MR. *The Joy of Cooking.* Indianapolis: Bobbs-Merrill Company, Inc.; 1975.

6. Winter R. *Super Soy: The Miracle Bean.* New York: Crown
    Trade Paperbacks; 1996.
7. Greenberg P. *The Whole Soy Cookbook.* New York: Three
    Rivers Press; 1998.
8. Messina M, Messina V, Setchell K. *The Simple Soybean and
    Your Health.* Garden City Park, NY: Avery Publishing Group;
    1994.

ADDITIONAL RESOURCES

The following organizations provide useful information about menopause and health issues related to midlife and aging (modified from *Menopause Guidebook*, North American Menopause Society, 1999).

COMPREHENSIVE INFORMATION

American College of Obstetricians and Gynecologists Resource Center (ACOG)
P.O. Box 96920
Washington, DC 20090-6920
www.acog.com

No calls; send a self-addressed, stamped envelope.

American Society for Reproductive Medicine (ASRM)
209 Montgomery Highway
Birmingham, AL 35216
205-978-5000
www.asrm.com

Booklets available for a nominal charge.

Association of Women's Health, Obstetric and Neonatal
  Nurses (AWHONN)
2000 L Street, NW, Suite 740
Washington, DC 20036
202-261-2400
800-673-8499
www.awhonn.org

National Association for Professionals in Women's Health
  (NAPWH)
175 West Jackson Boulevard, A1711
Chicago, IL 60604
312-786-1468
www.napwh.org

Call or write for referrals to women's health-care centers in your
  area.

National Women's Health Network
514 10th Street, NW, Suite 400
Washington, DC 20004
202-628-7814

Call or write for free information.

The North American Menopause Society (NAMS)
P.O. Box 94527
Cleveland, OH 44101
440-442-7550
800-774-5342
(automated line for consumers)
www.menopause.org

Call or write for free "MenoPak" containing booklet plus a
   suggested reading list and a list of menopause clinicians and
   discussion groups (nominal shipping/handling fee).

**The Society of Obstetricians and Gynecologists of Canada
   (SOGC)**
774 Echo Drive
Ottawa, ON K1S 5N8
613-730-4192
www.medical.org

Educational information available on Web site, or through the
   Osteoporosis Society of Canada.

CANCER

American Cancer Society
800-ACS-2345
www.cancer.org

Call for free literature.

Canadian Breast Cancer Foundation
790 Bay Street, Suite 1000
Toronto, ON M5G 1N8
800-387-9816 (Canada only)

Canadian Cancer Society
10 Alcorn Avenue, Suite 200
Toronto, ON M4V 3B1
416-961-7223

888-387-9816
www.cancer.ca

Cancer information service for Canada only.

Gynecological Cancer Foundation
401 N. Michigan Avenue
Chicago, IL 60611-4267
800-444-4441

Call or write for free booklets.

CANCER INFORMATION HOTLINE

National Cancer Institute
800-422-6237 (800-4-CANCER)

Call for free information.

HEART DISEASE

American Heart Association
7272 Greenville Avenue
Dallas, TX 75231-4567
214-373-6300
800-AHA-USA1
www.americanheart.org

Call or write for free information.

The Heart and Stroke Foundation of Canada
222 Queen Street, Suite 1402

Ottawa, ON K1P 5V9
613-569-4361
888-473-4636 (Canada only)
www.hsf.ca

Call or write for free literature.

National Heart, Lung, and Blood Institute
9000 Rockville Pike
Building 31, Room 4A-21
Bethesda, MD 20892
301-251-1222
800-575-WELL

Call for recorded messages on cardiovascular disease, or write
   for free facts on heart disease.

STOPPING SMOKING

American Lung Association
140 Broadway
New York, NY 10019
212-315-8700
800-LUNG-USA
www.lungusa.org

Call or write for free literature.

MENTAL HEALTH

American Psychological Association
750 First Street, NE
Washington, DC 20002

800-374-2721
www.apa.org

Call or write for free literature or referrals.

Canadian Mental Health Association
2160 Yonge Street, 3rd Floor
Toronto, ON M4S 2Z3
416-484-7750
www.icomm.ca-cmhacan

Call or write for free referrals to local branches.

National Institute of Mental Health Literature
5600 Fishers Lane
Public Inquiries Office
Room 7C-02
Mailing Code MSC 8030
Bethesda, MD 20892
301-443-4513
www.nimh.nih.gov

Call or write for free literature.

OSTEOPOROSIS

National Osteoporosis Foundation (NOF)
1150 17th Street, NW, Suite 500
Washington, DC 20036
800-223-9994
www.nof.org

Call or write for free literature.

Osteoporosis Society of Canada
P.O. Box 280
Station Q
Toronto, ON M4T 2M1
416-696-2663
800-977-1778 (Canada only, French)
800-463-6842 (Canada only, English)

Call or write for free information (Canada only).

SEXUAL ISSUES

**Sexuality Information and Education Council of the U.S.
  (SIECUS)**
130 West 42nd Street, Suite 350
New York, NY 10036
212-819-9770
www.siecus.org

Call or write for free literature.

UROGENITAL CONDITIONS

Interstitial Cystitis Association
P.O. Box 1553
Madison Square Station
New York, NY 10159
212-979-6057
www.ichelp.com

Call or write for a free brochure.

National Association of Incontinence
P.O. Box 8310
Spartanburg, SC 29305
800-BLADDER
www.nasc.org

Call for free information.

National Vulvodynia Association
P.O. Box 4491
Silver Spring, MD 20914-4491
301-299-0775
www.nva.org

Call or write for free brochure/national support network
information.

The Simon Foundation for Incontinence
P.O. Box 835
Wilmette, IL 60091
800-23-SIMON

P.O. Box 66524
Cavendish Mall P.O.
Cote St. Luc, PQ H4W 3J6
800-265-9575 (Canada only)

Call or write for free information packet.

The Vulvar Pain Foundation
P.O. Box 177
Graham, NC 27253
336-226-0704
www.vulvarpainfoundation.org

Write for information (nominal postage fee).

GENERAL INFORMATION ON SOY

Here are knowledgeable sources for additional information about soy.

American Soybean Association
540 Maryville Centre Drive, Suite 390
St. Louis, MO 63141
314-576-1770

Free information and recipes.

Archer Daniels Midland (ADM) Corporation
Box 1470
Decatur, IL 62525
800-637-5850

Largest producer of soy products in the United States.

Indiana Soybean Board
423 West South Street
Lebanon, IL 46052-2461
800-825-5769

Publishes U.S. Soy Foods Directory.

National Soybean Research Laboratory (NSRL)
University of Illinois at Urbana-Champaign
170 Environmental and Agricultural Sciences Building
1101 West Peabody Drive
Urbana, IL 61801
217-244-1706

Publishes three bulletins per year.

Ohio Soybean Council
Two Nationwide Plaza
P.O. Box 479
Columbus, OH 43216-1479
614-249-2492

Soyfoods Center
P.O. Box 234
Lafayette, CA 94549
510-283-2991

Provides information on soy and soy products.

United Soybean Hotline
6000 West Executive Drive
P.O. Box 249
Mequon, WI 53092
800-825-5769

Soy recipes, health, and agricultural information.

INDEX

Page numbers in *italics* refer to illustrations.